S0-AWO-275

Go For FIT

THE WINNING
WAY TO
FAT LOSS

What others say about Sherri Kwasnicki:

"Sherri Kwasnicki is a leader in the personal training field and a worthy recipient of IDEA's first Personal Trainer of the Year Award."
— Kathie Davis, Executive Director, IDEA: The Health & Fitness Source

"Sherri has a real knack for taking cumbersome concepts and breaking them down into understandable chunks of information. She does a tremendous job of educating everyday people about the importance of healthy living by giving them real life solutions to common wellness challenges. Her sense of humour and down to earth sincerity make her a top fitness educator and author, for both fitness professionals and the consumer."
— Sharon Donaldson, Association Director, Can-Fit-Pro

"Sherri is creative, energetic and inspirational. In addition to all the positive and practical things you will get from reading this book, you will learn that life is meant to be enjoyed. Sherri has an appreciation of life that is infectious!"
— Maureen Hagan, National Director of Fitness, The GoodLife Fitness Clubs

"Go For Fit is the first honest, realistic book on achieving the quality of life we all seek. Sherri gives us gold medal tools to reach our comfortable fitness levels and feel good about ourselves. She is our mentor-coach; we become our own personal trainer. It's a winning formula."
— Diane Clement and Doug Clement, M.D.

"Sherri's experience and knowledge as a fitness trainer is extensive. She combines a good, solid common-sense approach with scientific knowledge and proven principles of exercise. In addition, Sherri's understanding of how to motivate people has really helped me to achieve and maintain my health goals."
— Rick Hansen

Go For FIT

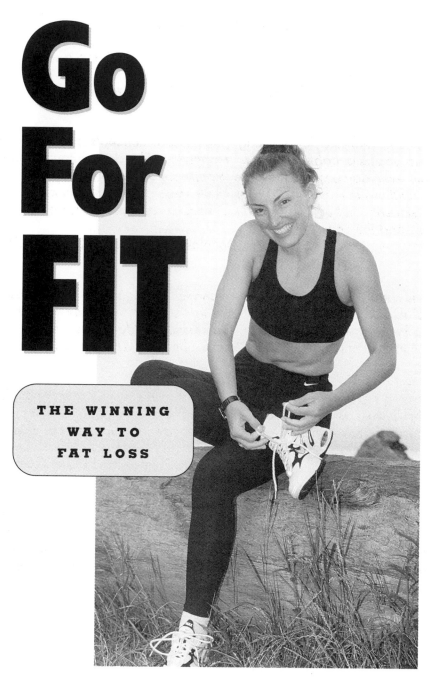

THE WINNING WAY TO FAT LOSS

SHERRI KWASNICKI

M.Sc.

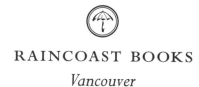

RAINCOAST BOOKS

Vancouver

DEDICATION

To the Hegmans and the rest of my family: You've always been there for me, no matter what!

Text copyright©1999 by Sherri Kwasnicki
Photographs© 1999 by John Darch

All rights reserved. No part of this publication may be reproduced or transmitted in any
form or by any means, electronic or mechanical, including photocopying, recording or by
any information storage and retrieval system, now known or to be invented,
without permission in writing from the publisher.

First published in 1999 by

Raincoast Books
8680 Cambie Street
Vancouver, B.C.
V6P 6M9
(604) 323-7100

Web site: www.raincoast.com

1 2 3 4 5 6 7 8 9 10

CANADIAN CATALOGUING IN PUBLICATION DATA

Kwasnicki, Sherri.
Go for fit

ISBN 1-55192-264-9

1. Exercise.   2. Reducing diets.   3. Physical fitness.   I. Title.
RA781.6.K82 1999   613.7   C99.910496-9

Printed in Canada

Editing by Paper Trail Publishing
Text design by Inklings Design

Raincoast Books gratefully acknowledges the support of the Government of Canada,
through the Book Publishing Industry Development Program, the Canada Council
and the Department of Canadian Heritage. We also acknowledge the assistance of the
Province of British Columbia, through the British Columbia Art Council.

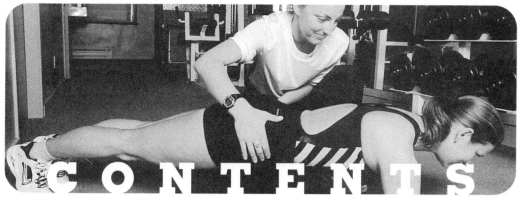

CONTENTS

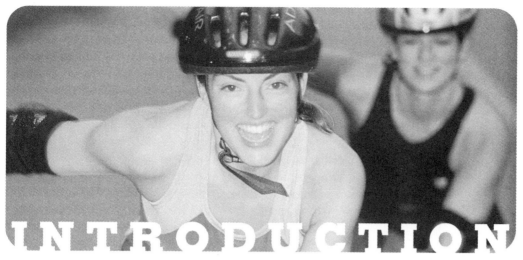

INTRODUCTION

go for FIT

We as a population are much more educated about fitness and nutrition than we were a few decades ago. We know that we should be exercising and eating well. And healthier food is much more accessible. So why is our population, both adults and children, continuing to get fatter? According to the National Center for Health Statistics in the United States, the average adult weighs eight pounds (3.6 kg) more than they did a decade ago. And did you know that 32 percent of men and 35 percent of women are considered not just overweight but obese? Here is another scary statistic: the average 154-pound (70-kg) male gains 22 pounds (10 kg) of fat in 20 years. That is a pound a year! We're not going to look so hot at the high-school reunion, are we?

These statistics have to concern us. Obesity is associated with an increased risk of hypertension, diabetes, cardiovascular disease and many cancers. We have to consider its effects on our joints and our backs, not to mention its psychological effects on our self-esteem and confidence.

For as long as I can remember, I have noticed that people who were active or played sports always seemed to be able to do more things, always had more fun. They just seemed to be able to enjoy life more than their sedentary, unfit counterparts. Fit people generally do not smoke, so they are less likely than smokers to get cancer. They generally don't carry a lot of excess body fat so they suffer fewer heart attacks than those who are unfit. Fit people have stronger lungs, muscles, joints and bones. Their immune systems are healthier, as are their hearts. Their cholesterol levels and blood pressure measurements are better.

By now you can see how passionate I am about the benefits of exercise. I honestly believe that if everybody on earth were exercising regularly, we could expect to enjoy world peace. Think about it! If people were exercising regularly, they would probably have less time to get into fights. I also find that people who exercise regularly tend not to get as upset about the little things; it is almost as if the energy they are

> DREAMING HAS ITS PLACE; INSPIRATION IS INVALUABLE; BUT LIFE IS ACTION AS WELL AS THOUGHT. THEY GET FARTHEST IN THE REALM OF CHARACTER-BUILDING WHO LINK UP THOUGHT AND ACTION, WHO DO NOT MERELY DREAM, BUT ACT UPON THEIR NOBLEST IMAGININGS.
>
> R.W. WILDE

expending helps them to burn off excess anger or frustration. I think we should consider writing to our politicians to suggest they cut the defence budget and spend the money on getting the 80 percent of our population that is sedentary hooked on exercise. I think we would notice a huge difference in many of our societal problems.

Our growing weight problem can be attributed to many factors. One, we do not move as much as we used to. The *International Journal of Obesity* estimates that we expend 500 to 800 fewer calories per day than we did 30 years ago. Modern transportation, escalators, elevators, computers and remote controls are all helping us to pack on the pounds. Secondly, the majority of us still have not gotten the message about the importance of exercise. Eighty percent of our population does not exercise regularly or vigorously enough to obtain any health benefits. And, finally, our food portion sizes have increased dramatically. We are suffering from the trend of "supersizing." Oversize cookies, fries, shakes, muffins and bagels are adding calories to our diets without us noticing. These three factors have caused the rate of obesity to rise so that it is quite visible on our streets. Spend an afternoon people-watching in a major North American city and you will quickly see the effects of our new culture.

If one of us does decide we would like to lose some weight, we know pretty much what we need to do. The information is out there for us in abundance. It is not like we would think, "Exercise?! Is that what I need to do to lose weight?" or "Eat healthier to lose weight?! Why didn't I think of that?" No, we know exactly what we need to do. In fact, we have no problem initiating the process. We have done it numerous times. We tend to lose fat over and over again. The problem – and our struggle – lies in the challenge of keeping the weight off. Most people who undertake a fat loss program have not really taken the time to fully understand the complexity of the process. They have examined only the physiology or the science of fat loss and have neglected the psychological and behavioural-change aspects. If you are going to succeed at initiating these major changes in your life and, more importantly, maintaining the changes, you are going to have to establish a very strong foundation for success. You will have to do your homework.

Once you decide you need to lose body fat, you generally have a few options. You might decide, like most people, to diet. Unfortunately, the research is conclusive and indicates that diets do not work, with 98 percent of people gaining the weight back.

Or you might decide to exercise. Although exercise on its own is a very healthy choice, most people find it too slow a process and give up before they start to experience the benefits. If you were to start an exercise program now without modifying your diet, you could expect a two-percent change in your body fat over a 12- to 18-week period. This would equate to three pounds (1.4 kg) of fat lost, and although this is a significant change, when, like most people, you want to lose 10 pounds (4.5 kg) by the weekend, the process is painfully slow. Most people start to measure their effort and compare it to the results. Many have a difficult time justifying their five-times-a-week exercise program when the end result is one pound (0.45 kg) lost per month. In fact, studies demonstrate that seven out of 10 people who start an exercise program quit within the first three months. And most do so because they have not seen the results they were expecting.

There is also, of course, the really quick approach to fat loss – liposuction. But although liposuction works to remove some of the unwanted fat cells, if you do not change your lifestyle habits and start exercising and eating well, the fat cells that you still have will just get bigger and you will not be any better off – just a few thousand dollars poorer.

There are hundreds of fat loss books on the shelves. I remember my publisher asking me, "What is going to be so different about your fat loss book?" I answered confidently, "This book is going to make a difference. People are actually going to get results!" With most books, you read them and then they go back on the bookshelf. By the time you start to initiate any of the changes, you have forgotten what they were in the first place and you have probably lost the motivation anyway. This book is an interactive book. You will regularly be asked to take action toward your goals. You will be asked to answer questions, complete homework drills, sign a Fat Loss Contract and keep a Daily Exercise and Nutrition Log. This will force you to implement the information immediately and to keep your goals front and foremost.

This workbook will enable you to examine the physiology of fat loss – the cold, hard facts. You will be given the tools to understand how the physiology and the psychology of fat loss can work very closely together to ensure your success. You will examine your thoughts, feelings and negative patterns. You will establish realistic and positive goals and outline obstacles that may surface and strategies for overcoming them. And you will learn the most effective exercise and nutrition tips for maximizing safe, effective and permanent fat loss. You will be your own personal trainer – designing your own program, monitoring your progress and modifying the program along the way. You will be captain of your own ship. I will only be the guide.

The health and fitness industry is now quite convinced that the safest and most effective program for permanent fat loss is one that combines exercise and a healthy diet. This workbook will focus on that combination. I am a firm believer that there is no quick fix. Expect to put forth a bit of effort. You know what they say: "If something is worth having, it is worth working for." Completing this workbook is not going to be a cakewalk, but I can guarantee you that it is probably not going to be as difficult as you imagine.

Every drill in this book will take you closer to success. Every homework assignment you complete will give you the confidence and self-esteem to know you can accomplish the next goal. It is all about "results momentum." If I ask you to do something, even if it is a really small task, and you do it, you have succeeded. This will give you momentum, and reaching the next goal will become that much easier. If you do not do the task, no matter how insignificant, you will find it easier to skip out on other tasks – maybe ones that are much more important to your success. So think of this process as a series of baby steps, with each taking you closer and closer to permanent fat loss.

If I have not yet convinced you of the merits of a healthy diet and exercise, let me ask you this. When you are 70 years old, would you rather be confined to a rocking chair in a nursing home or out hiking the mountains, cross-country skiing through the woods, kayaking the oceans and playing with your grandkids? It is your choice. If you are not enjoying the life or the body you want now or when you are older, you have no one to blame but yourself.

Let's get started right away. Why wait till you finish the book? Good luck! Remember, I have full confidence that you can do this because I know that "If you think you can, you can."

Sherri

ACKNOWLEDGEMENTS

As with any piece of work, there are numerous people who have provided support, feedback and guidance. They all deserve recognition.

I would like to express my extreme gratitude to the team at Raincoast Books. It's been a joy to work with each of you. Special thanks go to Brian Scrivener, who approached me to write this book. If it weren't for you, Brian, I'd probably still just be *thinking* about writing this book.

I'd also like to say thanks to my teachers and role models who have, collectively, provided me with the knowledge, tools, and experiences to present this material to you: Len Kravitz, Matt Church, Daniel Kosich, Wayne Westcott, Allan Martin, Rich Hansen, Peter and Kathie Davis, David Patchell-Evans and Maureen Hagan.

I'd also like to thank *The Province* newspaper, *Chatelaine* and *Go!* Magazines and other trade journals and publications for allowing me the opportunity to write and develop my skills so that I could competently finish this book.

To Sandy Boucher, my client, friend and model for the photographs in this book: Sandy, thanks for your patience and upbeat, positive attitude. Thanks also to John Darch, our photographer, who was so generous with his time and talents.

And finally, to those who are close to me, my friends, family and clients, who support me unconditionally in all my ambitious — thanks for your love.

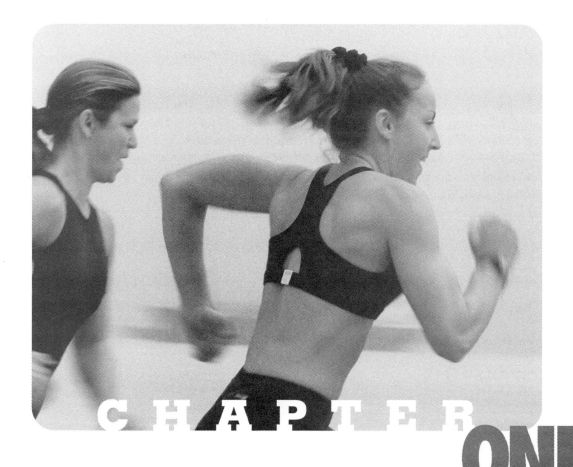

CHAPTER ONE

THE PSYCHOLOGY OF FAT LOSS

OVERCOMING NEGATIVE THOUGHTS

There is more to fat loss than you might think. Fat loss is a complex psychological phenomenon and can often result in a vicious cycle of weight loss and weight gain. Once we make a conscious decision to drastically reduce our caloric intake, we instantly experience deprivation. This often results in feelings of anger as we question why others can eat Häagen-Dazs and chocolate and not struggle with their weight. Our willpower slowly dwindles, and inevitably we give in to one of our temptations. We feel like a failure and decide, since we have screwed up, we might as well "go for the gusto" and binge on all our favourite foods. Afterwards, we feel out of control and guilty for our actions. We feel hopeless and desperate and turn to food to comfort us. This just fuels our insecurities and low self-esteem, as we start to believe we are fat, ugly and a loser. We decide the only way to feel better is to lose the weight, and the cycle starts again.

Part of initiating a fat loss program is understanding the psychology of our behaviours and actions. There are lots of things we can do to gain control of our actions. One aspect of gaining control is understanding the role of negative and irrational thinking. We are often our own worst critics and can be very hard on ourselves. Here are some things you might have said to yourself that might have sabotaged your fat loss efforts in the past.

- *I missed my workout. The whole day is ruined. I am a total loser!*
- *If I do not starve myself, I will get fat.*
- *Since I pigged out at lunch, the whole day is ruined. I might as well stuff myself today and start all over again tomorrow.*
- *Things always go wrong. I am such a failure!*
- *It is not the diet program that is wrong, it is me!*
- *I might have lost 10 pounds, but I cannot go to the beach until I am a perfect size 6.*
- *I will be happy once I lose weight.*
- *My thighs are the fattest I have ever seen!*
- *If I look like Kate Moss, then my boyfriend will pay more attention to me.*
- *Why do I have so little willpower?*
- *Why couldn't I just have been born with a perfect body?*
- *I have to lose 20 pounds within a month to get ready for my vacation or my holidays will be ruined!*
- *I must never eat anything fattening.*
- *These things always happen to me.*
- *I will always be like this.*
- *I can't seem to do anything right.*
- *Why would anybody love me?*

MANY WISE SAYINGS EXPRESS THE EFFECTS OUR THINKING HAS ON OUR BEHAVIOURS

"What concerns me is not the way things are, but rather the way people think things are."

EPICTETUS

"Energy follows thought. You actually become what you think."

LYNNE NAMKA

"Change your thoughts and you change your world."

NORMAN V. PEALE

"Negative thinking will always lead to failure; but positive faith – positive thinking – will lead you towards happy, healthy and abundant living."

ALBERT E. CLIFFE

"If you realized how powerful your thoughts are, you would never think a negative thought. They can have a powerful influence for good when they're on the positive side, and they can and do make you physically ill when they're on the negative side."

PEACE PILGRIM

"Once you understand the basic irrational beliefs you create to upset yourself, you can use this understanding to explore, attack, and surrender your other present and future emotional problems."

ALBERT ELLIS

We cannot take our thoughts lightly, because they can directly affect our actions and our progress. However, there *are* things that we can do immediately to overcome or control negative or irrational thinking. Here are some tips.

> WHEN YOU LOVE
> WHO YOU ARE,
> THERE IS NOTHING
> UNCONQUERABLE,
> NOTHING
> UNREACHABLE.
>
> RAMTHA

1. Listen to your thoughts at the times when you feel worst.

2. Listen for irrational or negative thinking.

3. Dispute these thoughts by asking, "Why is this so? Where is this negativity coming from?" and "Could there be another possible explanation or interpretation?"

4. Imagine repeating what you have said to a close friend or child. We could never imagine talking to others as we often talk to ourselves. The next time you catch yourself thinking irra-tionally or negatively, ask yourself if you would ever speak this way to another human being. You deserve the same type of respect you would give anybody else! Remind yourself that if you continually practise negative self-talk, eventually you might start to believe your own words. Your self-esteem can end up taking a real beating.

5. Displace irrational thoughts by techniques such as:

   • **Thought stopping.** *When worrying, instantly think of a stop sign, then focus on pleasant thoughts.*

   • **Stress management.** *When worrying, participate in your favourite relaxation techniques, such as massage, reading, baths, journal writing, etc.*

   • **Thought reversal.** *Have positive messages or quotes posted around your workplace or home to help you put things into perspective.*

6. Learn to live in the moment and to experience true joy in your life. Stop worrying about the past or the future. Most people have a very difficult time living in the now. Try this easy drill. Shut your eyes. Listen and try to identify all the sounds around you. Smell for different scents. Open your eyes and really look around you. Observe all the different colours and objects. The next time you eat, try to eat slowly and taste every single bite. Quick drills like this will help you to develop the skill of living in the moment.

7. Each night before you fall asleep, make a mental note of the best part of your day or of something you experienced that you really appreciated or enjoyed. By doing this, you will learn to look for the good things in life.

8. Live today! Self-hatred takes a lot of time and energy. Obsessing about your body weight, nutrition plan and exercise program can leave you tired and depressed. Deciding to not enjoy the here and now because you have decided to wait until you lose weight will leave you feeling deprived and will often lead to more negative feelings and behaviours. Remember that thin thighs, a small butt and a six-pack set of abdominals are not the ticket to a meaningful existence. Fill your life with interesting experiences and people and you will enjoy a much higher quality of life.

It is now time to put this information to good use. Answer the following questions to help identify negative or irrational thoughts that you might experience. I suggest you use a pencil throughout this workbook.

1. What negative or irrational thoughts have you experienced in the past? (Do you call yourself names? Do you establish unrealistic expectations? Do you constantly point out the negatives?)

_____

_____

_____

_____

_____

_____

_____

_____

_____

_____

_____

_____

_____

_____

2. What are some different explanations to dispute these irrational or negative thoughts?

_____

_____

_____

_____

_____

_____

_____

_____

_____

_____

_____

_____

_____

_____

3. What can you and are you willing to do to change
these thoughts?

_____

_____

_____

_____

_____

_____

_____

_____

_____

_____

_____

_____

_____

_____

_____

_____

_____

_____

_____

_____

_____

_____

_____

_____

_____

THE BODY AND
THE MIND ARE SO
CLOSELY CONNECTED
THAT NOT EVEN A
SINGLE WORD OR
THOUGHT CAN
COME INTO
EXISTENCE WITHOUT
BEING REFLECTED
IN THE PERSONALITY
AND HEALTH
OF THE
INDIVIDUAL.

JOHN
PRENTISS

4. This next drill will help you to form new positive thoughts and perceptions. Write a positive, supportive, loving letter to yourself. The letter should include all the things you love about yourself. You should write about all the things that make you special – the things you are proud of. Include a section that discusses all the wonderful things you are going to do for yourself. Tell yourself that because you love yourself so much you are going to, for example, be more active, eat a more healthy diet, get a massage once a month, get eight hours of sleep every night, surround yourself with positive people . . .

_____

_____

_____

_____

_____

_____

_____

_____

_____

_____

_____

_____

_____

_____

_____

_____

_____

_____

_____

_____

_____

_____

_____

_____

_____

_____

_____

_____

> TO EFFECTIVELY CHANGE YOURSELF, YOU MUST BELIEVE YOURSELF CAPABLE OF CHANGING AND YOU MUST HAVE NO BELIEFS WHICH PREVENT THAT CHANGE.
>
> PAUL E. WOOD

An old habit is hard to break. As humans, we are creatures of habit, and we often do things not because we need to but simply because we have always done them. Some common examples are:

- *salting our food*

- *eating during commercials*

- *always purchasing food at the movies*

- *eating while studying*

- *always overeating at parties*

- *snacking while making dinner*

- *eating poorly when we are with friends*

- *always eating the same amount of food, regardless of our hunger level*

- *stopping for an ice-cream cone or treat on our way home from a weekend destination, regardless of our hunger level*

The movies just would not be the same without popcorn. This is a habit, and often people find themselves ordering popcorn even though they have just had dinner and are feeling quite satisfied. Another example is the midway rest stop when coming home from the cottage or a weekend ski trip. People get into the habit of stopping for a Dairy Queen Blizzard™ or another favourite treat regardless of their hunger level. Students often get into the habit of eating while studying for exams.

The first step to getting control of these dietary habits is to become aware of your patterns. In this workbook you will fill out a Daily Exercise and Nutrition Log that will allow you to track your behaviours. The log will make patterns and habits very obvious. Once you discover what stimulates your less-than-healthy behaviour, you can choose to either (a) change the stimulus or situation or (b) change your *response* to the stimulus or situation.

Here are the active steps you can take to overcome habitual dietary behaviours.

Step 1. Recognize what stimulates the unhealthy action. Become aware of the habit. Monitor what you eat, when you eat, who you are with and how you felt.

Step 2. Change the stimulus.

Step 3. Change the response.

HOMEWORK

FOR EXAMPLE:

UNHEALTHY BEHAVIOUR	CHANGE STIMULUS	CHANGE RESPONSE
Whenever you are depressed, you eat junk food.	Try not to get overly depressed. Instead, examine whether there could be any positive outcomes from the depressing situation. Try to develop the skills to become optimistic.	When you get depressed, watch a funny movie or call a best friend or go for a long walk.
Whenever you go out with Patti, you always drink too much and eat terribly .	When you go out with Patti, bring along another friend who might be a better influence.	You and Patti make a healthy dinner at home and then go out dancing, both agreeing that you will drink two glasses of water for every beer or alcoholic drink.
Every Friday night, friends come over to watch a rental movie and you always eat eight slices of pizza.	Instead of watching a movie, schedule a hike or a walk with your friends.	Order Japanese food instead of pizza.
Every time you eat ice cream, you always order a double scoop.	Instead of ordering ice cream, order a fruit salad.	Order one scoop of ice cream instead of two.
You always eat two sandwiches at lunch.	Bring a bowl of chili to lunch.	Eat one sandwich and a small salad.
You always go to the cafeteria and buy two chocolate chip cookies for your mid-afternoon break.	Take a short walk on your break instead.	Bring a few fruit or fig bars to work for your break.

1. List the dietary stimulants and responses you participate in regularly.

_____

_____

_____

_____

_____

_____

_____

_____

_____

_____

_____

_____

_____

_____

2. What actions can you take to overcome these connections and change your behaviour?

_____

_____

_____

_____

_____

_____

_____

_____

_____

_____

_____

_____

_____

People often have very unrealistic expectations about the type of body they would like to achieve. They sometimes refer to popular magazines for an image of their ideal body. But they ignore the fact that many of the models are 23 percent underweight, some have had "body-enhancing" surgery and they have spent hours being made up. Camera tricks are used, and once the photos have been developed, the pictures are cropped, airbrushed and manipulated by computer to produce an unrealistic, unhealthy and so-called perfect image.

It is very important for you to examine your genetics and to understand that fat loss is dependent on your genetic background. Approximately 40 percent of "fatness" is genetically determined. You cannot change this! It's also important to note the differences between being overfat and being overweight. Some thin, sedentary people can be underweight and overfat. Others, such as a football player, can be overweight and have a normal amount of body fat. Obesity is a term I will use to refer to those who carry enough body fat to be considered at risk for many health complications. Regardless, genetics play an important role that should not be overlooked. Here are some statistics to help you understand this relationship.

If one of your parents is obese, you are twice as likely to be overfat. If both of your parents are obese, you are four times as likely to be overfat. One study makes this relationship very clear. Overfat sets of identical twins were fed 1,000 extra calories per day for seven weeks. You would expect all of the twins to gain exactly the same amount of weight, but, in fact, the weight gain ranged from 9.5 to 29.3 pounds (4.3 to 13.3 kg). And although the range of weight gain was wide, the twins in each pair gained exactly the same amount of weight.

Here is the message. You do have a choice. If you are a pear-shaped individual, you can choose to be an in-shape pear shape or an out-of-shape, fatter pear shape, but you are always going to be a pear shape. So examine your parents and other members of your family to determine the types of expectations you should have.

What I find sad are the men and women who get caught in the "Geez, if I could just lose this extra 10 pounds, then I'd be happy" syndrome, yet when they do lose the weight, are still not satisfied. If you believe that you will be happy once you lose weight, you will never be skinny enough to be happy. It is a vicious cycle, and it never ends unless we learn to love the body we have as it is right now – not tomorrow or next month or next year.

It is okay to want to make health improvements, but you cannot hate and despise the state you are in now. Making these lifestyle changes is about believing you deserve to be healthier! You deserve to take the time out to exercise and eat well. It is not about making the changes so you can look like someone else. If you make changes with the latter as your ultimate goal, you will not succeed and you will be miserable for life. Take my word for it. I have seen it happen time and time again. Body hatred and dissatisfaction are hardly reserved for the morbidly obese. Many women who clearly have very little body fat to lose are not happy with their body proportions. Take control of your happiness today!

Did you know that the average North American woman is five foot four (1.6 m), weighs 140 pounds (63.5 kg) and wears a size 14 dress? Yet the "ideal" woman portrayed by models and movie stars is five foot seven (1.7 m), weighs 100 pounds (45.3 kg) and wears a size 8. What is wrong with this picture?

Body dissatisfaction is at an all-time high among both men and women. Check out the following startling facts.

- *Seventy-five percent of women are dissatisfied with their appearance. Of those, 89 percent say they want to lose weight. Twenty-two percent of men say they want to gain weight. In general, men are more satisfied with their appearance than women, although the number of men who are tormented about their weight and shape is climbing.*

- *Fifteen percent of women and 11 percent of men, respectively, say they would sacrifice more than five years of their life to be the ideal weight, while 24 percent of women and 17 per cent of men say they would give up more than three years.*

- *Fifty percent of women are on a diet at any given time.*

- *The weight loss industry (diet foods, programs and drugs) takes in more than $40 billion each year and continues to grow.*

- *Young girls are more afraid of becoming fat than they are of nuclear war, cancer or losing their parents.*

- *Fifty percent of nine-year-old girls and 80 percent of 10-year-old girls have dieted.*

- *Anorexia has the highest mortality rate (up to 20 percent) of any psychiatric illness.*

- *Girls are more prone to developing eating and self-image problems than to developing drug or alcohol problems. Yet there are drug and alcohol programs in almost every school but very few eating disorder programs.*

- *One to two percent of women between the ages of 14 and 25 have anorexia; three to five percent experience bulimia; and another 10 to 20 percent of women in this age group engage in many of the behaviours associated with both eating problems.*

I sincerely hope these statistics, released by various eating disorder organizations, have scared you into examining your own body image issues and have caused you to consider how you could improve upon your own beliefs.

HOMEWORK

Step 1. Decide what's a realistic body type for you. Answer the following questions to help separate fact from fantasy.

1. Is there a history of excess fat in your family?

_____

_____

_____

_____

_____

2. Which parts of your body or physical attributes are you satisfied with?

_____

_____

_____

_____

_____

_____

_____

_____

_____

3. What is the lowest weight you have maintained as an adult for at least one year?

_____

_____

_____

4. Based on your genetic predisposition, your age and the amount of time you want to spend exercising, what type of physique is achievable for you? This should be your "ideal."

_____

_____

_____

_____

_____

_____

_____

_____

_____

_____

_____

Step 2. Realize that your past does not equal your future. Traumatic things that might have happened to you in your past, such as sexual, physical or verbal abuse, significantly influence your present perception of yourself. It is imperative that you re-create your body image by recognizing and releasing these feelings from the past.

1. Make a time line of the events in your life that you believe contributed to your body image. Start with childhood memories and continue to the present. What types of messages did your parents give you about your body? How did other relationships affect your body image?

_____

_____

_____

_____

_____

_____

_____

_____

_____

_____

_____

_____

_____

_____

_____

_____

_____

_____

_____

_____

_____

_____

_____

_____

_____

_____

_____

_____

_____

2. List all the things you can do to take care of yourself and your body. What actions can you take on a regular basis to demonstrate that you love yourself and that you deserve to be healthy?

_____

_____

_____

_____

_____

_____

_____

_____

_____

_____

_____

_____

_____

Step 3. Get a little help from your friends. Surround yourself with positive, supportive people who are part of the solution, not part of the problem.

1. List the people you would like to surround yourself with because you know they will be positive and supportive of your ambitions.

_____

_____

_____

_____

_____

_____

2. Make a mental note of the people you will spend less time with because you feel they might be a negative influence.

Now that you have realistically analyzed your thoughts, feelings, habits and genetics, you are prepared to approach fat loss with a more positive perspective. You may find it necessary and helpful to come back to this chapter and perform the drills regularly when you find yourself resorting to old, negative thought patterns or behaviours.

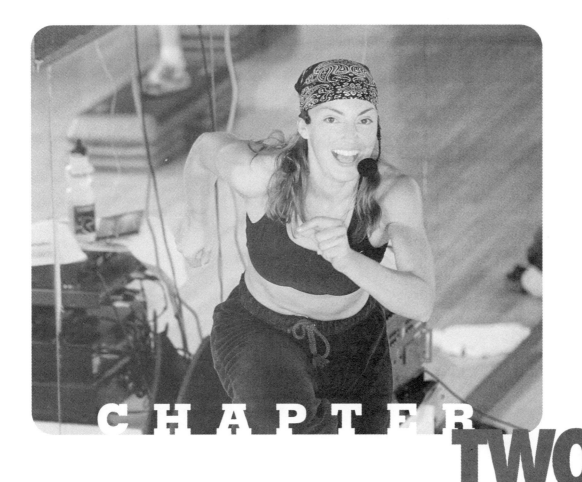

CHAPTER TWO

USE THE SCALE AND PLAN TO FAIL

If we are going to measure your success, we are going to need appropriate and correct indicators of progress. Unfortunately, most people make their biggest mistake in this area. They measure their fat loss success by jumping on the scale. They think that if they have lost weight, they have succeeded; if not, they have failed. But it is not that simple. If you use the scale as your only indicator of success, you are setting yourself up for failure.

Imagine you have been exercising for a whole week and watching your food intake. Then you step onto the scale and find your weight has not changed or, heaven forbid, it has actually increased. But the scale tells you only one thing – your total body weight in pounds or kilograms. It does not tell you anything about how much of that weight is comprised of muscle, bone, fat or water.

Have you heard that muscle weighs more than fat? Wrong. One pound of muscle weighs the same as one pound of fat – one pound (0.45 kg). But a pound of muscle is more dense than a pound of fat, so it takes up a lot less space. Think of a rock that weighs one pound and a feather pillow that weighs one pound. By the same token, a 140-pound (63.5-kg) woman who carries a lot of muscle will look very different from a woman of the same weight who carries very little muscle. She will appear smaller and leaner than her less-muscled counterpart, even though they weigh exactly the same.

Imagine you begin an exercise and nutrition program that causes you to lose a few pounds of body fat – a positive change. If, however, you are following a sensible exercise program, you will also have begun a resistance training program, which could cause you to gain three to four pounds of lean tissue after eight to 12 weeks. The end result will be no change in your body weight, and you will think whatever you are doing is not working very well. But, your body will have undergone positive changes that will have put you on the right path to weight loss. You see, muscle is an energy-burning tissue, and the more muscle you carry on your body, the easier it is for you to expend calories both at rest and during exercise.

Relying on the scale to measure fat loss is inappropriate for a number of other reasons.

- *Body weight can fluctuate by several pounds throughout the day.*
- *You could be retaining water and misinterpret the weight gain as body fat gain.*
- *Women experience large weight fluctuations due to hormonal changes during their menstrual cycles.*
- *After you eat, your weight increases.*

Here is a chart of the results that can be seen in an exercise and nutrition program. It demonstrates why weight loss is not a good measure of success.

SAMPLE RESULTS

	BASELINE	AFTER 3 MONTHS	VARIATION
Body weight	133.7 pounds (60.6 kg)	134.7 pounds (61.1 kg)	+ 1.0 pound (+ 0.45 kg)
Body fat %	28%	25%	- 3%
Fat weight	35.9 pounds (16.3 kg)	32.9 pounds (14.9 kg) - 3.0 pounds	- 3.0 pounds (- 1.4 kg)
Lean-tissue weight	97.8 pounds (44.4 kg)	101.8 pounds (46.2 kg)	+ 4.0 pounds (+ 1.8 kg)

The scale may show little change in weight, but the scale shows only part of the picture. To get the whole picture, and to see changes that show your program is working, you'll need three other indicators: body measurements, Polaroid shots and a subjective measurement of how clothing fits. For example, wouldn't you be pleased to know that although your weight hadn't changed, you had in fact dropped inches in all your measurements, you appeared leaner in your Polaroid shots and you could tighten your belt by two notches?

If you are going to use the scale as one of your indicators of success, you should weigh yourself on the same scale each time and ensure that the scale has not been tampered with or adjusted between measurements. I also recommend that you weigh yourself only once per month, then put the scale away. I would hate for you to be discouraged by a scale reading that misrepresents the true picture.

MEASURING YOUR BODY

Body measurements are one method of monitoring your progress, but I caution against using them alone. When muscle gain occurs more rapidly than fat loss, the end result is larger measurements and utter frustration. You can take comfort in knowing that these larger measurements will not be permanent and if you stay focused on your program, the measurements will eventually start to get smaller. The same situation can happen if you decide to measure your progress using the fit of your clothes. You may at one point feel your clothes getting tighter rather than looser. Be persistent.

> ONE DAY AT A TIME – THIS IS ENOUGH. DO NOT LOOK BACK AND GRIEVE OVER THE PAST, FOR IT IS GONE; AND DO NOT BE TROUBLED ABOUT THE FUTURE, FOR IT HAS NOT YET COME. LIVE IN THE PRESENT, AND MAKE IT SO BEAUTIFUL THAT IT WOULD BE WORTH REMEMBERING.
>
> IDA SCOTT TAYLOR

HOMEWORK

You can go to a gym and hire a personal trainer or go to a laboratory and pay for an expensive, high-tech fitness assessment. But that is not necessary. You can get all the information you need to measure your progress in the privacy of your own home. Okay, it is time to determine your baseline measurements. I believe in examining the entire picture and thus encourage you to use as many of the tools as possible. This will give you a much better picture of your progress. Here are some guidelines.

- *Acquire the services of a close friend, family member, partner or personal trainer to assist you with these measurements. This person should agree to support you throughout the entire process, because you will need them to measure you a number of times. The accuracy of the results is improved if the same person measures you each time.*

OUR FATE IS
MATCHED BY
THE TOTAL
FREEDOM WE
HAVE TO REACT
TO OUR FATE.
IT IS AS IF
WE WERE DEALT
A HAND OF
CARDS. ONCE
WE HAVE THEM,
WE ARE FREE
TO PLAY
THEM AS WE
CHOOSE.

THOMAS
SOWELL

- *Ensure that you have not consumed caffeine, alcohol or drugs 24 hours prior to an assessment, because they might affect your hydration levels and the accuracy of the measurements.*

- *Measure yourself in the morning, before you have exercised.*

- *Wear clothing that is minimal and revealing to ensure accurate measurements. A bathing suit or underwear is recommended.*

- *Refer to the following notes in this chapter to ensure precision in all measurements.*

- *Record exactly where on your body you measured the first time to ensure later measurements are taken in exactly the same spot. Even if you are off by less than one inch (2.5 cm), the discrepancy could dramatically affect the result.*

- *Complete the form titled Success Assessment: Baseline Test. Complete a retest form once per month for the first three months. After this, measuring yourself every three to six months should be adequate.*

Measure the following sites:

Chest: I recommend both a mid-chest and an upper-chest measurement. The upper-chest measurement is taken by placing the tape under the armpits and measuring the chest circumference at that level. For women, the upper-chest measurement does not include the breast tissue. The mid-chest measurement for men is right across the nipple line. For women, the mid-chest measurement is the largest circumference around the breast and includes the breast tissue.

Abdomen: I suggest three measurements of this area: the upper waist, waist and lower waist. The upper-waist measurement is usually taken about two inches (5 cm) above the navel; you can measure at any point, depending on your body dimensions, as long as you record exactly how high above the navel you measured. The waist measurement is taken at the navel. The lower-waist measurement is taken approximately two inches (5 cm) below the navel; but again, you can measure at any point as long as you record exactly how low below the navel you measured. For women, the lower-waist measurement is usually the largest abdominal circumference.

Hips: Position the measuring tape at the point where your buttocks protrude. The hip measurement is the circumference of the hips at their widest point.

Thighs: I encourage two measurements for the thighs: upper and mid thigh. For the upper thigh, measure closer to the crotch at the level on the thigh where the buttocks end and the thigh begins. For the mid thigh, take the measurement midway up the thigh. Eyeball this point, but then be sure to record exactly how high above the kneecap you measured to ensure the reliability of future measurements.

To calculate your **waist-to-hip ratio,** take your waist measurement and divide it by your hip measurement. The result gives you a rough indicator of your fat distribution. For example, if your waist measured 31.5 inches (80 cm) and your hips measured 39.4 inches (100 cm), your waist-to-hip ratio would be 0.8. Some studies have concluded that a ratio greater than 0.8 in women and greater than 1.0 in men indicates an increased risk for cardiovascular disease. A lower waist-to-hip ratio suggests a reduced risk for cardiovascular disease.

The last and most helpful tool in monitoring fat loss success is a Polaroid picture. A photo leaves nothing to be misinterpreted. It reveals quite obviously if and where someone has been losing body fat.

If you decide to use Polaroid shots, you must wear minimal clothing to be able to see any significant changes. You must ensure that the person taking the shots stands exactly the same distance away from you each time, and you need to wear exactly the same articles of clothing each time to ensure you are not deceived by colour or cut. I also encourage you to have three shots taken: one from the front, one from the side and one from the back.

Now complete the Success Assessment Form.

BODY FAT PERCENTAGE

Should you be wondering about your body fat percentage, assessment tools are readily available. Underwater weighing, skinfold calipers, bioelectrical analysis and others all claim to measure body fat percentages accurately. However, you should be cautioned that the science of body fat assessment is infested with error. In my undergraduate studies in kinesiology, my professor demonstrated this point by having each of us measure our body fat percentage using a number of different measuring tools. On that day, my body fat varied from seven percent to 28 percent, depending on the measuring tool.

Each tool has its own vulnerabilities. Underwater weighing is the present gold standard for body fat measurement. Most other techniques have been developed in correlation to the results from underwater weighing. Each technique thus holds it own sources of error and is also affected by the errors associated with underwater weighing. The end result is an inexact science.

Although I use skinfold measurements to monitor success with my clients, instead of calculating body fat percentages, I add all the skinfold measurements to obtain a total. If the sum drops, fat loss is indicated and I know we are going in the right direction. You, too, can perform skinfold measurements in your success assessment, but because body fat assessment tools require expert assistance, I have not described how to use them. If you do decide you want this information included in your baseline measurements, I encourage you to have a local personal trainer perform the test(s) for you.

> TO TAKE A JOURNEY OF A THOUSAND MILES, YOU HAVE TO BEGIN WITH THE FIRST STEP FROM THE PLACE WHERE YOU STAND; THE ROMANTIC DESCRIPTION OF THE JOURNEY AND THE THINGS THE BODY SEES ON THE WAY AND THE DESCRIPTION OF THE SCENERY ARE OF NO USE UNLESS YOU LIFT YOUR FOOT AND TAKE THE FIRST STEP.
>
> VIMALA THAKAR

SUCCESS ASSESSMENT

BASELINE TEST

Date: _____ **Time of day:** _____

Special considerations or circumstances:

_____

_____

_____

Complete only one column: imperial or metric

	IMPERIAL	METRIC
Weight	pounds	kg
Upper chest	inches	cm
Mid chest	inches	cm
Upper waist (_____ above waist)	inches	cm
Waist	inches	cm
Lower waist (_____ below waist)	inches	cm
Hips	inches	cm
Upper thigh	inches	cm
Mid thigh (_____ above kneecap)	inches	cm
Waist-to-hip ratio		
Polaroid shot (_____ away from camera)		

CLOTHING NOTES: *Comment on the tightness of a notched belt you are presently using. Comment on the magnitude and location of tightness of a particular outfit.*

_____

_____

_____

_____

_____

SUCCESS
ASSESSMENT

RETEST 1

Date: _____   **Time of day:** _____

Special considerations or circumstances:

_____

_____

_____

	IMPERIAL	METRIC	CHANGE +/−
Weight	pounds	kg	
Upper chest	inches	cm	
Mid chest	inches	cm	
Upper waist (_____ above waist)	inches	cm	
Waist	inches	cm	
Lower waist (_____ below waist)	inches	cm	
Hips	inches	cm	
Upper thigh	inches	cm	
Mid thigh (_____ above kneecap)	inches	cm	
Waist-to-hip ratio			
Polaroid shot (_____ away from camera)			

CLOTHING NOTES: *Comment on the tightness of a notched belt you are presently using. Comment on the magnitude and location of tightness of a particular outfit.*

_____

_____

_____

_____

_____

SUCCESS ASSESSMENT

RETEST 2

Date: _____   **Time of day:** _____

Special considerations or circumstances:

_____

_____

_____

	IMPERIAL	METRIC	CHANGE +/−
Weight	pounds	kg	
Upper chest	inches	cm	
Mid chest	inches	cm	
Upper waist (_____ above waist)	inches	cm	
Waist	inches	cm	
Lower waist (_____ below waist)	inches	cm	
Hips	inches	cm	
Upper thigh	inches	cm	
Mid thigh (_____ above kneecap)	inches	cm	
Waist-to-hip ratio			
Polaroid shot (_____ away from camera)			

CLOTHING NOTES: *Comment on the tightness of a notched belt you are presently using. Comment on the magnitude and location of tightness of a particular outfit.*

_____

_____

_____

_____

_____

SUCCESS ASSESSMENT

RETEST 3

Date: _____ **Time of day:** _____

Special considerations or circumstances:

_____

_____

_____

	IMPERIAL	METRIC	CHANGE +/−
Weight	pounds	kg	
Upper chest	inches	cm	
Mid chest	inches	cm	
Upper waist (_____ above waist)	inches	cm	
Waist	inches	cm	
Lower waist (_____ below waist)	inches	cm	
Hips	inches	cm	
Upper thigh	inches	cm	
Mid thigh (_____ above kneecap)	inches	cm	
Waist-to-hip ratio			
Polaroid shot (_____ away from camera)			

CLOTHING NOTES: *Comment on the tightness of a notched belt you are presently using. Comment on the magnitude and location of tightness of a particular outfit.*

_____

_____

_____

_____

_____

SUCCESS ASSESSMENT

RETEST 4

Date: _____   **Time of day:** _____

Special considerations or circumstances:

_____

_____

_____

	IMPERIAL	METRIC	CHANGE +/−
Weight	pounds	kg	
Upper chest	inches	cm	
Mid chest	inches	cm	
Upper waist (_____ above waist)	inches	cm	
Waist	inches	cm	
Lower waist (_____ below waist)	inches	cm	
Hips	inches	cm	
Upper thigh	inches	cm	
Mid thigh (_____ above kneecap)	inches	cm	
Waist-to-hip ratio			
Polaroid shot (_____ away from camera)			

CLOTHING NOTES: *Comment on the tightness of a notched belt you are presently using. Comment on the magnitude and location of tightness of a particular outfit.*

_____

_____

_____

_____

_____

SUCCESS ASSESSMENT

R E T E S T   5

Date: _____   **Time of day:** _____

Special considerations or circumstances:

_____

_____

_____

	IMPERIAL	METRIC	CHANGE +/−
Weight	pounds	kg	
Upper chest	inches	cm	
Mid chest	inches	cm	
Upper waist (_____ above waist)	inches	cm	
Waist	inches	cm	
Lower waist (_____ below waist)	inches	cm	
Hips	inches	cm	
Upper thigh	inches	cm	
Mid thigh (_____ above kneecap)	inches	cm	
Waist-to-hip ratio			
Polaroid shot (_____ away from camera)			

CLOTHING NOTES: *Comment on the tightness of a notched belt you are presently using. Comment on the magnitude and location of tightness of a particular outfit.*

_____

_____

_____

_____

_____

CAN YOU LOSE TOO MUCH BODY FAT?

It is important to realize that it is possible to lose too much body fat. Some of the unhealthy symptoms are:

- *loss of energy or feeling tired*
- *feeling unusually irritable*
- *immune system suppression (always getting sick or injured)*
- *dry, itchy skin; brittle hair*
- *loss of menstrual cycle*
- *people's negative or concerned comments about your health and appearance*

If you notice one or more of these symptoms, you should examine your exercise and nutrition program to ensure you are not expending too much energy and ingesting too few calories. You should also immediately consult with your physician to examine your situation and adjust your program.

HOW FIT IS YOUR HEART?

You might want to test your cardiovascular fitness at the outset of your fat loss program. Visit your doctor and have her check out your heart. Here's a simple assessment you can do very easily at home. Map out a distance – let's say, three miles (4.8 km) -then walk or jog it. Time yourself. As your heart and lungs get fitter, you will be able to perform the same distance in a shorter period of time. Alternatively, you could assess your cardiovascular fitness on a treadmill, a stationary bike or a rowing machine.

HOMEWORK

Perform this assessment at your earliest convenience and complete the following chart.

CARDIOVASCULAR ASSESSMENT

	BASELINE TEST 1	TEST 2	TEST 3	TEST 4
Date				
Activity				
Distance				
Time				

HOW FIT ARE YOUR MUSCLES?

The fitness of your muscles is very easy to measure on an ongoing basis. When you are performing certain exercises, as you are able to lift more weight or perform more repetitions, you can be confident that your muscles are getting stronger. For example, if you can lift a five-pound (2.3-kg) hand weight 15 times at the beginning of your program and, two months later, you can lift a 10-pound (4.5-kg) hand weight 15 times, your strength has improved by 100 percent. Or if you can perform 10 push-ups when you start and, a month later, you can do 20 push-ups, your muscular endurance is definitely improving.

HOW FIT IS YOUR BLOOD PRESSURE?

People who exercise have healthier blood pressures than those who don't. You might find it helpful to include a blood pressure test in your success assessment. An at-home blood pressure machine can be purchased for about $40. Many physicians encourage their patients to purchase these machines, because the home is a more comfortable environment than the doctor's office, and you can test yourself more regularly. You can also monitor your blood pressure at some pharmacies.

LOVE HANDLES AND BIG THIGHS

It doesn't take a rocket scientist to figure out that men and women deposit their body fat differently. Men tend to store all their fat around their abdominal region, and women store it in their hips and thighs. Remember that lovely saying "A moment on the lips, a lifetime on the hips"? Well, for women, it holds a bit of truth.

Elite-level female runners carry very little body fat, yet when you look at pictures of them, you can clearly see that many still have very stubborn and resistant thigh fat. Some even have cellulite! Even though most women struggle with it, this type of fat distribution is in fact much healthier than male fat distribution. The fat in women's hips and thighs is very resistant to reduction (don't we know!), but this female fat distribution is less of a strain on the heart, and there is a smaller chance that the fat will be deposited in the artery walls. For men, however, their distribution of fat is a double-edged sword. Their abdominal fat is much more responsive, so that once they start exercising and eating better, they often lose fat more quickly than women. But if they are not exercising, the excess abdominal fat causes the heart to work a lot harder. And if the muscles are not using the fat, it is more likely to be deposited in the artery walls, increasing the risk of heart disease. Your waist-to-hip ratio will help you keep track of the distribution of your body fat and its implications for your health. Remember a lower waist-to-hip ratio will suggest a lower risk of heart disease.

SPOT REDUCING DOES NOT WORK

This is probably a good time to quickly debunk any persistent beliefs about spot reduction. Ladies, 1,000 leg lifts are not going to help you get rid of the fat on your thighs. And gentlemen, 1,000 crunches are not going to help you get rid of your pot belly. Advertisements promising localized fat reduction infuriate fitness professionals, who know that what is being promised is impossible. What happens, say, during leg lifts is that as soon as you start, your muscles cry out for energy. But there is no direct line from the muscle cells to the fat cells surrounding them. So your liver sends some energy, in the form of sugar or fat, to the muscle being used. But that fat might have come from your arm, butt or back. When fat is mobilized from a particular area, it is first sent to the liver to be routed toward its final destination for usage. So doing leg lifts does not mean you are burning leg fat. If your leg fat is very resistant to mobilization, which it is in most women, then it will be stubborn and probably will be the last fat to be mobilized and utilized. As you exercise regularly, you will likely notice great changes to your arms and stomach and other areas and start to wonder when your lower body fat is going to start cooperating. Be patient; losing this fat is just going to take longer. Doing specific body part exercises will definitely help to tone muscle, but unfortunately, you cannot "spot reduce" fat. If you want to see a reduction in fat in a particular area, you are going to have to exercise and eat a healthy diet. And, of course, you'll need patience for those stubborn areas.

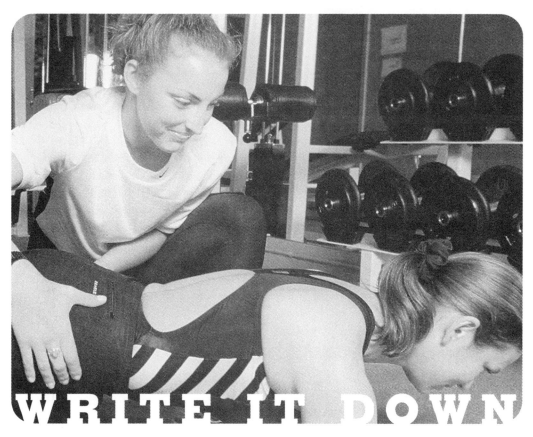

WRITE IT DOWN

SIGNING YOUR FAT LOSS CONTRACT & KEEPING A DAILY EXERCISE & NUTRITION LOG

Now it's time to put it in writing – affirming your commitment in a Fat Loss Contract and recording your progess in a daily log. The purpose of this contract is to serve as a reminder to you of the commitment to a healthy lifestyle that you have made to yourself. You have made one of the best decisions of your life. You might consider having someone you trust witness this contract to further support you as you persevere towards your goals.

Studies have shown that just the act of recording your exercise and the foods you eat instantly and significantly results in healthier choices. A journal can also reveal bad habits or patterns you have developed. For example, you might notice that on the days you exercise, you eat well, and the days you do not, your nutrition is poor. In this fat loss workbook, I expect you to keep a Daily Exercise and Nutrition Log on an ongoing basis. Complete the forms at the end of each day. Be as detailed as possible, using the following instructions as a guide.

Here is what you will be required to track in your log on a daily basis.

1. **Exercise.** Record exactly how much cardiovascular and muscle-conditioning exercise you perform each day, as well as the intensity of each workout and the type of exercise.

2. **Nutrition.** Record precisely *when* you eat or drink anything. You might notice that you consistently eat too late, that most of your calories are consumed too late in the day, that you are eating too few meals or that you are leaving too much time between meals. Look for unhealthy patterns. Record exactly *what* you eat and drink. This data is very important, and it needs to be precise. It helps if you carry your logbook with you so you can record your meal right after you eat. You should record every single thing you put in your mouth –

HE WHO

MOVES

NOT

FORWARD

GOES

BACKWARD.

JOHANN W.

GOETHE

including water – and record the exact amounts. Noting portion size is critical to helping you determine where you can cut back if you need to reduce your caloric intake. Record *where* you eat and who you are with. You might notice that when you sit in front of the TV you always eat or eat too much. You might discover that on the weekends when you go out with friends, you always overeat. You might determine you are a social eater. Record how you feel *during* each meal. Are you bored, lonely, depressed, excited, happy, stressed out? You might discover that you are an emotional eater and need to come up with a list of alternative activities for times when you are experiencing these feelings. Record how you feel *after* each meal. Did you overeat or did you eat just until you were comfortably satisfied?

3. Daily gratification. I like to include a section in the daily log where I record at least one thing that happened or something I saw on that day that I am grateful for. It just seems to add so much more value to each and every day. I find that then I am always looking for the positive in life instead of simply "giving in" to the stresses and daily turmoils.

4. Goal setting. I like to encourage setting and reassessing goals on a daily basis. Every day, decide what your goal for the day will be, whether it is drinking eight glasses of water, eating five vegetable servings or consuming five small meals instead of three big ones. Pick an area from Your Fat Loss Contract that you need to focus on, then stick with it for the entire day. At the end of the day reassess your goal. Did you achieve it? If you did, congratulations! If not, why not? What can you do tomorrow to ensure success? You can reset the same goal or focus on a completely different area.

At the end of each week, complete the Weekly Synopsis sheet. This sheet gives you an overview of how you did throughout the previous week. It will help you determine which areas you are succeeding in and which areas require greater focus. You will require a calculator to perform the synopsis.

I have included one week of Daily Exercise and Nutrition Logs. I suggest you keep a master copy and go to your local print shop and make more copies. Just the act of tracking your progress on a long-term basis will help keep you on your program.

HOMEWORK

1. Review and sign the following Fat Loss Contract. Have a witness sign also.

2. Go to your local print shop and print eight copies (for eight weeks) of your Exercise and Nutrition Logs (plus the Weekly Synopsis). Keep the master copy in a safe place.

3. Tonight, before bed, throughly complete Day One of your Exercise and Nutrition Log.

YOUR FAT LOSS CONTRACT

Review the following list. This is an overview of some of the basic steps you can start to take immediately to help maximize fat loss. I will explain the reasoning behind these expectations later in this book. But rather than waiting to read the entire book, start on some of these goals right away. You will be that much further ahead. You might even see noticeable, visible improvements by the time you complete this book! There are 11 things you must commit to in order to achieve your goals in a safe, effective and permanent fashion. You can choose to focus on just a couple or tackle all of them at once.

1. You must exercise aerobically five to seven days each week for 20 to 60 minutes each session. You must exercise at an intensity that gets you breathing and sweating, at a perceived exertion rating of five to eight (see page 91). Activities such as walking, jogging, cycling, swimming, rowing, stair climbing or fitness classes will do the trick.

2. You must condition your muscles with resistance training workouts two times per week. One set of eight to 12 repetitions of a variety of exercises is sufficient.

3. You must eat three small meals and two snacks each day.

4. You must eat five vegetable servings and three fruit servings each day.

5. You must drink eight glasses of water each day.

6. You must limit your alcohol intake or eliminate it from your diet.

7. You must stop eating three hours before bedtime.

8. You must make a commitment to maintaining a more active daily lifestyle.

9. You must be sure to get enough sleep.

10. You must control your stress levels.

11. You must complete your Daily Exercise and Nutrition Log every day.

_____

I promise to follow the above prescription to the best of my ability.

Date: _____   Signed: _____

Date: _____   Witness Signature: _____

DAILY EXERCISE & NUTRITION LOG

DAY ONE

DATE: _____

1. EXERCISE

CARDIOVASCULAR	MUSCLE-CONDITIONING
Time: Intensity: Type:	Time: Intensity:

2. NUTRITION

BREAKFAST	MID-MORNING SNACK	LUNCH	MID-AFTERNOON SNACK	DINNER
Time: What: Location/ Environment: Feelings:	Time: What: Location/ Environment: Feelings:	Time: What: Location/ Environment: Feelings:	Time: What: Location/ Environment: Feelings:	Time: What: Location/ Environment: Feelings:

Did you drink eight glasses of water today?

YES   **NO**   How many? _____

Did you eat five vegetable servings today?

YES   **NO**   How many? _____

Did you eat three fruit servings today?

YES   **NO**   How many? _____

Did you eat five small meals or snacks today?

YES   **NO**   How many? _____

Did you drink any alcohol today?

YES   **NO**   How much? _____

Did you stop eating two to three hours before bed?

YES   **NO**   When? _____

> **BELIEVE YOU CAN AND YOU CAN. BELIEVE YOU WILL AND YOU WILL. SEE YOURSELF ACHIEVING, AND YOU WILL ACHIEVE.**
>
> **GARDNER HUNTING**

Comment on your mood/energy/psychological state today:

_____

_____

_____

3. Today I am grateful for:

_____

_____

_____

4. My major accomplishment(s) today were:

_____

_____

_____

Were today's goals achieved?   **YES**   **NO**

Tomorrow's goal(s) will be:

_____

_____

_____

_____

_____

DAILY EXERCISE & NUTRITION LOG

DAY TWO

DATE: _____

1. EXERCISE

CARDIOVASCULAR	MUSCLE-CONDITIONING
Time: Intensity: Type:	Time: Intensity:

2. NUTRITION

BREAKFAST	MID-MORNING SNACK	LUNCH	MID-AFTERNOON SNACK	DINNER
Time: What: Location/ Environment: Feelings:	Time: What: Location/ Environment: Feelings:	Time: What: Location/ Environment: Feelings:	Time: What: Location/ Environment: Feelings:	Time: What: Location/ Environment: Feelings:

Did you drink eight glasses of water today?

YES   **NO**   How many? _____

Did you eat five vegetable servings today?

YES   **NO**   How many? _____

Did you eat three fruit servings today?

YES   **NO**   How many? _____

Did you eat five small meals or snacks today?

YES   **NO**   How many? _____

Did you drink any alcohol today?

YES   **NO**   How much? _____

Did you stop eating two to three hours before bed?

YES   **NO**   When? _____

THE GREAT
END OF LIFE
IS NOT
KNOWLEDGE,
BUT
ACTION.

THOMAS
FULLER

Comment on your mood/energy/psychological state today:

_____

_____

_____

3. Today I am grateful for:

_____

_____

_____

4. My major accomplishment(s) today were:

_____

_____

_____

Were today's goals achieved?   **YES**   **NO**

Tomorrow's goal(s) will be:

_____

_____

_____

_____

_____

DAILY EXERCISE & NUTRITION LOG

DAY THREE

DATE: _____

1. EXERCISE

CARDIOVASCULAR	MUSCLE-CONDITIONING
Time:	Time:
Intensity:	Intensity:
Type:	

2. NUTRITION

BREAKFAST	MID-MORNING SNACK	LUNCH	MID-AFTERNOON SNACK	DINNER
Time: What:	Time: What:	Time: What:	Time: What:	Time: What:
Location/ Environment:	Location/ Environment:	Location/ Environment:	Location/ Environment:	Location/ Environment:
Feelings:	Feelings:	Feelings:	Feelings:	Feelings:

Did you drink eight glasses of water today?

YES   **NO**   How many? _____

Did you eat five vegetable servings today?

YES   **NO**   How many? _____

Did you eat three fruit servings today?

YES   **NO**   How many? _____

Did you eat five small meals or snacks today?

YES   **NO**   How many? _____

Did you drink any alcohol today?

YES   **NO**   How much? _____

Did you stop eating two to three hours before bed?

YES   **NO**   When? _____

THE RESULT
OF ANY ACTION
IS DEPENDENT
UPON THE
AMOUNT OF
CONFIDENCE
WITH WHICH
IT IS
DONE.

SATHYA
SAI BABA

Comment on your mood/energy/psychological state today:

_____

_____

_____

3. Today I am grateful for:

_____

_____

_____

4. My major accomplishment(s) today were:

_____

_____

_____

Were today's goals achieved?   **YES**   **NO**

Tomorrow's goal(s) will be:

_____

_____

_____

_____

_____

DAILY EXERCISE & NUTRITION LOG

DAY FOUR

DATE: _____

1. EXERCISE

CARDIOVASCULAR	MUSCLE-CONDITIONING
Time:	Time:
Intensity:	Intensity:
Type:	

2. NUTRITION

BREAKFAST	MID-MORNING SNACK	LUNCH	MID-AFTERNOON SNACK	DINNER
Time:	Time:	Time:	Time:	Time:
What:	What:	What:	What:	What:
Location/ Environment:	Location/ Environment:	Location/ Environment:	Location/ Environment:	Location/ Environment:
Feelings:	Feelings:	Feelings:	Feelings:	Feelings:

Did you drink eight glasses of water today?

YES   **NO**   How many? _____

Did you eat five vegetable servings today?

YES   **NO**   How many? _____

Did you eat three fruit servings today?

YES   **NO**   How many? _____

Did you eat five small meals or snacks today?

YES   **NO**   How many? _____

Did you drink any alcohol today?

YES   **NO**   How much? _____

Did you stop eating two to three hours before bed?

YES   **NO**   When? _____

Comment on your mood/energy/psychological state today:

_____

_____

_____

3. Today I am grateful for:

_____

_____

_____

4. My major accomplishment(s) today were:

_____

_____

_____

Were today's goals achieved?   **YES**   **NO**

Tomorrow's goal(s) will be:

_____

_____

_____

_____

_____

> BAD TIMES
> HAVE SCIENTIFIC
> VALUE. THESE
> ARE OCCASIONS
> A GOOD
> LEARNER WOULD
> NOT MISS.
>
> RALPH WALDO
> EMERSON

DAILY EXERCISE & NUTRITION LOG

DAY FIVE

DATE: _____

1. EXERCISE

CARDIOVASCULAR	MUSCLE-CONDITIONING
Time: Intensity: Type:	Time: Intensity:

2. NUTRITION

BREAKFAST	MID-MORNING SNACK	LUNCH	MID-AFTERNOON SNACK	DINNER
Time: What: Location/ Environment: Feelings:	Time: What: Location/ Environment: Feelings:	Time: What: Location/ Environment: Feelings:	Time: What: Location/ Environment: Feelings:	Time: What: Location/ Environment: Feelings:

Did you drink eight glasses of water today?

     YES   **NO**   How many? _____

Did you eat five vegetable servings today?

     YES   **NO**   How many? _____

Did you eat three fruit servings today?

     YES   **NO**   How many? _____

Did you eat five small meals or snacks today?

     YES   **NO**   How many? _____

Did you drink any alcohol today?

     YES   **NO**   How much? _____

Did you stop eating two to three hours before bed?

     YES   **NO**   When? _____

> DON'T TAKE YOURSELF SO SERIOUSLY. LAUGH AND PLAY. IT'S NOT THE END OF THE WORLD IF SOMETHING DOESN'T GO RIGHT.
>
> SANAYA ROMAN

Comment on your mood/energy/psychological state today:

_____

_____

_____

3. Today I am grateful for:

_____

_____

_____

4. My major accomplishment(s) today were:

_____

_____

_____

Were today's goals achieved?   **YES**   **NO**

Tomorrow's goal(s) will be:

_____

_____

_____

_____

_____

DAILY EXERCISE & NUTRITION LOG

DAY SIX

DATE: _____

1. EXERCISE

CARDIOVASCULAR	MUSCLE-CONDITIONING
Time:	Time:
Intensity:	Intensity:
Type:	

2. NUTRITION

BREAKFAST	MID-MORNING SNACK	LUNCH	MID-AFTERNOON SNACK	DINNER
Time:	Time:	Time:	Time:	Time:
What:	What:	What:	What:	What:
Location/ Environment:	Location/ Environment:	Location/ Environment:	Location/ Environment:	Location/ Environment:
Feelings:	Feelings:	Feelings:	Feelings:	Feelings:

Did you drink eight glasses of water today?

YES   **NO**   How many? _____

Did you eat five vegetable servings today?

YES   **NO**   How many? _____

Did you eat three fruit servings today?

YES   **NO**   How many? _____

Did you eat five small meals or snacks today?

YES   **NO**   How many? _____

Did you drink any alcohol today?

YES   **NO**   How much? _____

Did you stop eating two to three hours before bed?

YES   **NO**   When? _____

> WE ARE LIVING
> IN A WORLD
> OF BEAUTY,
> BUT FEW OF
> US OPEN
> OUR EYES
> TO SEE IT.
>
> **LORADO
> TAFT**

Comment on your mood/energy/psychological state today:

_____

_____

_____

3. Today I am grateful for:

_____

_____

_____

4. My major accomplishment(s) today were:

_____

_____

_____

Were today's goals achieved?   **YES**   **NO**

Tomorrow's goal(s) will be:

_____

_____

_____

_____

_____

DAILY EXERCISE & NUTRITION LOG

DAY SEVEN

DATE: _____

1. EXERCISE

CARDIOVASCULAR	MUSCLE-CONDITIONING
Time: Intensity: Type:	Time: Intensity:

2. NUTRITION

BREAKFAST	MID-MORNING SNACK	LUNCH	MID-AFTERNOON SNACK	DINNER
Time: What:	Time: What:	Time: What:	Time: What:	Time: What:
Location/ Environment:	Location/ Environment:	Location/ Environment:	Location/ Environment:	Location/ Environment:
Feelings:	Feelings:	Feelings:	Feelings:	Feelings:

Did you drink eight glasses of water today?

YES　　　　**NO**　　　　How many? _____

Did you eat five vegetable servings today?

YES　　　　**NO**　　　　How many? _____

Did you eat three fruit servings today?

YES　　　　**NO**　　　　How many? _____

Did you eat five small meals or snacks today?

YES　　　　**NO**　　　　How many? _____

Did you drink any alcohol today?

YES　　　　**NO**　　　　How much? _____

Did you stop eating two to three hours before bed?

YES　　　　**NO**　　　　When? _____

> ANYTIME YOU SINCERELY WANT TO MAKE A CHANGE, THE FIRST THING YOU MUST DO IS RAISE YOUR STANDARDS.
>
> **ANTHONY ROBBINS**

Comment on your mood/energy/psychological state today:

_____

_____

_____

3. Today I am grateful for:

_____

_____

_____

4. My major accomplishment(s) today were:

_____

_____

_____

Were today's goals achieved?　　　**YES**　　　　**NO**

Tomorrow's goal(s) will be:

_____

_____

_____

_____

_____

WEEKLY SYNOPSIS

WEEKLY SYNOPSIS	ACTUAL	GOAL
1. Total cardiovascular time (minutes)		> 100 min.
2. Total number of cardio sessions		5 to 7
3. Total number of muscle-conditioning workouts		2
4. Average number of glasses of water per day		8
5. Average number of vegetable servings per day		5
6. Average number of fruit servings per day		3
7. Number of days five small meals or snacks consumed		7
8. Number of days alcohol was consumed		0 to 1
9. Number of days stopped eating three hours before bed		7

Major accomplishment(s) this week:

_____

_____

Next week's goal(s):

_____

_____

_____

_____

_____

_____

_____

_____

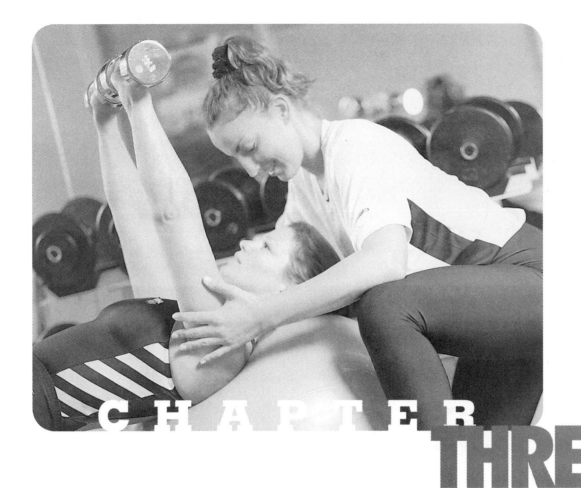

CHAPTER THREE

BEHAVIOURAL
CHANGE

As a personal trainer, I have interacted with clients who succeed easily and others who struggle tremendously. The sad fact is that seven out of 10 people who start an exercise or nutrition program drop out within a few months. If you have been one of those seven in the past, the problem might not have been with you – it might have been with the method.

Most people attempt to do too much too quickly. They do not do any planning, and they have no idea how to monitor their progress. Your chances for success will improve dramatically if you plan your program, monitor your progress and break down the process into four separate steps.

Step 1. Determine how ready you are to make the changes.

Step 2. Develop concrete motivation for adhering to your program.

Step 3. Set SMART goals.

Step 4. Outline potential obstacles to success and strategies for overcoming them.

IN MANY
CASES STRESS
IS CAUSED NOT
BY THE EVENT
ITSELF BUT
RATHER BY OUR
RESPONSE TO
THE EVENT.

ROBERT

ELLIOT

Step 1. ARE YOU READY?

I generally know within a few minutes whether a client will succeed easily or not. If the client accepts my recommendations for changes to their exercise or nutrition program immediately and unconditionally, I know we will achieve success easily. If the client begins to make excuses or give reasons they feel they will not be able to adhere to the program, I can generally expect struggles throughout the process. They are not ready to make the changes required to see the results they want. I supply the following questionnaires to clients to help me determine where they are on the readiness scale. If they score poorly, I accept the fact that the timing might not be perfect for quick results. They can still initiate many of the changes and start to develop healthier habits, but I can expect some resistance to the changes. You can fill out the same questionnaires to determine how ready you are to initiate the lifestyle changes necessary to maximize fat loss.

HOMEWORK

Complete the following two questionnaires.

Readiness Questionnaire 1

1. Do you feel you are at some sort of health risk because of your current behaviours or lifestyle?	**YES**	**NO**
2. Do you feel that making lifestyle changes will improve your quality of life and decrease your risk of health-related disorders?	**YES**	**NO**
3. Do you view lifestyle change as a lifetime goal rather than a short-term temporary goal?	**YES**	**NO**
4. Are you willing to get personally involved in planning a lifestyle change program?	**YES**	**NO**
5. Are you willing to try different approaches?	**YES**	**NO**
6. Do you have the patience to accept success in small increments and deal with possible setbacks?	**YES**	**NO**
7. Are you willing to set realistic goals?	**YES**	**NO**
8. Are you willing to make lifestyle changes?	**YES**	**NO**

If you answered yes to all these questions, you are ready for action. If you said no to one or more of the questions, you might experience personal resistance as you initiate many of the actions required to achieve your fat loss goals. It might be helpful for you to review what is really important to you and learn more about the negative effects of your current behaviour and the benefits of change. Since preparation is crucial to your readiness to change, try the next questionnaire, too.

Readiness Questionnaire 2

1. Compared to previous attempts, how motivated are you this time to try to lose body fat?

| Not at all motivated | 1 | 2 | 3 | 4 | 5 | Extremely motivated |

2. How certain are you that you will stay committed to a fat loss program for the time it will take to reach your goal?

| Not at all certain | 1 | 2 | 3 | 4 | 5 | Extremely certain |

3. Considering all outside factors at this time in your life – the stress you are feeling at work, your family obligations, etc. – to what extent can you tolerate the effort required to stick to a lifetime exercise and nutrition plan?

| Cannot tolerate | 1 | 2 | 3 | 4 | 5 | Can tolerate easily |

4. Think honestly about how much weight you hope to lose and how quickly you hope to lose it. Figuring a healthy weight loss of one to two pounds per week, how realistic are your expectations?

| Very unrealistic | 1 | 2 | 3 | 4 | 5 | Very realistic |

5. Do you fantasize about eating your favourite foods?

| Always | 1 | 2 | 3 | 4 | 5 | Never |

6. How confident are you that you can work regular exercise into your daily schedule, starting tomorrow?

| Not at all confident | 1 | 2 | 3 | 4 | 5 | Extremely confident |

Score: 6-12: Low motivation   13-25: Moderate motivation   25+: High motivation

If you scored low, this might not be the best time for you to initiate major changes to your lifestyle. Such a score does not mean, however, that you cannot begin the program. You should just have lower expectations of yourself. If you scored moderately, expect a few struggles en route to your goals. If you scored high, this is the perfect time for you to begin taking action toward your goals. Good luck!

It is important to understand that change is a process. When initiating any major lifestyle change, you will experience the following stages. The entire process might take up to two years to complete.

1. Precontemplation. You have no intention of changing your behaviours.

2. Contemplation. You are aware a problem exists and are seriously thinking of changing.

3. Preparation. You are intending to take action in the next month and have unsuccessfully taken action in the past year.

4. Action. You are presently modifying your behaviour or environment.

5. Maintenance. You are working to prevent relapse and maintain your gains.

Do not be hard on yourself if you are having difficulty initiating action. Recognize where you are in the stages of change. Because you have purchased this book, you are probably at stage 2, 3 or 4. Don't be surprised, however, if you find yourself shifting between different stages. For example, many people attempt to stop smoking numerous times before they actually succeed. Do whatever you can to take action, and this will move you closer toward your goal. Purchasing this book was an active step that has already taken you closer to success.

HOMEWORK

1. Identify the stage of change you are in right now with regards to fat loss.

_____

_____

_____

_____

_____

_____

2. If you are in stages 1 to 3, what can you do to get yourself closer to taking action?

_____

_____

_____

_____

_____

_____

_____

_____

I have noticed a number of characteristics that separate those who succeed from those who do not. Those who succeed buy into the "Four Laws of Success." You must be ready to accept these laws without exception.

First Law: The law of possession. You need to understand that if you are going to achieve results, it is going to be up to you. The sayings "If it is going to be, it is up to me" and "If I think I can or think I can't, I'm right" ring very true. You have to take ultimate responsibility for success or failure. Sometimes I'll get a client who believes I am going to be the one who makes it happen for them. I set them straight right away. I tell them I cannot do anything for them. All I can do is educate and guide. They must be willing to make and stick to the changes. You cannot completely rely on someone else, such as a personal trainer or workout partner, to make it happen for you and, conversely, you cannot blame the kids or your partner for any failures.

Second Law: The law of effort. Anything worth achieving is worth working for. Exercise and healthy eating take discipline, willpower, character, persistence and a commitment to delayed gratification.

Third Law: The law of consistency. A month-long effort is not going to get you where you want to go. In order to achieve any goal, you must stick to your game plan on an ongoing, long-term, consistent basis. Getting off track for a week is no big deal if you are consistent in your efforts. But if you are regularly tempted away from your program, you will not succeed. Consistency and persistence are the keys to manifesting any goal. Remember that if you want to be 10 pounds (4.5 kg) thinner 10 years from now, it is not what you do over the next eight weeks that matters; it is what you do over the next 10 years. All the changes I will suggest must be followed for the rest of your life. They are not short-term, quick-fix solutions. Safe and permanent fat loss often takes years – not weeks or months.

Researchers have found only one characteristic common to those who succeed with exercise. All such people move toward their goal one step at a time. They are committed to constant, never-ending improvement. In practical terms, this means that regardless of anything else – busy work schedules, lack of energy, lack of time, feeling old, feeling lazy, hating exercise – they make no excuses. They keep exercising, taking their long-term goals and breaking them down into smaller goals. They take it one day at a time.

> HIGH ON THE WALL, IN THE CASTLE OF YOUR DREAMS OF SUCCESS, HANGS THE PICTURE OF WHAT YOU WANT TO BE. ALWAYS KEEP THAT PICTURE HANGING THERE. SEE YOURSELF WHERE YOU INTEND TO BE. NIGHT AND DAY DREAM OF WHAT YOU INTEND TO DO AND WHAT YOU INTEND TO BE, FOR YOUR DREAMS INTERPRET YOUR INTENTIONS ALWAYS. ALL SUCCESSES ARE, AT FIRST, DREAMS.
>
> FRED VAN AMBURGH

Fourth Law: The law of self-efficacy. If you are already questioning whether or not you can actually make the required changes, you are going to have a difficult time with your program. You must believe you can do it! Think of self-esteem as a bank. Each time you keep a promise to yourself, your store of self-esteem gets bigger, making it easier for you to keep the next promise to yourself. It's all about the "results momentum" I discussed earlier. Each time you break a promise, however, your self-esteem goes down, making it easier for you to break the next promise. Reinforce a belief in yourself by surrounding yourself with others who are doing or have accomplished what you're attempting. After all, if they can do it, so can you!

Step 2. ARE YOU MOTIVATED?

If you want to change something, you have to change something! Makes sense, doesn't it? But change is difficult. Most people attempt major changes in their life without setting up a framework for success. How can you get anywhere without a map or a game plan?

Finding the motivation and inspiration to maintain changes in your life day in, day out is challenging. Many people have very good intentions when they start an exercise or nutrition program, but within a few months the majority of them have dropped out. They could not find a reason to keep going. Much of being motivated boils down to associating pain with the situation you're in now – basically being "sick and tired of being sick and tired" – and associating pleasure with the situation you will be in once you achieve your goal. If you can develop these pain and pleasure sensations, you will pinpoint your personal motivation for exercise and healthy eating and you will find it much easier to stick with the program.

HOMEWORK

1. Write down all the pain you associate with being in your present situation. (For example, "None of my clothes fit. I have no energy. My blood pressure has risen. I can't sit comfortably in chairs. I feel embarrassed to wear a bathing suit.")

_____

_____

_____

_____

_____

_____

_____

_____

_____

_____

_____

2. Write down all the pleasure you associate with achieving your goals. (For example, "I'll be able to wear whatever I want. My energy level will improve. My blood pressure will drop. I'll be more productive at work. I'll feel more self-confident. I'll have enough energy to go hiking.")

_____

_____

_____

_____

_____

_____

_____

_____

_____

_____

_____

_____

> EVERYBODY IS UNIQUE. COMPARE NOT YOURSELF WITH ANYBODY ELSE LEST YOU SPOIL GOD'S CURRICULUM.
>
> **BAAL SHEM TOV**

Now go back and review your notes. Is there enough reason there for you to stick to your game plan no matter what? If not, go back and think more carefully. Maybe you will have to attach self-imposed pain to your present situation. For example, in Anthony Robbins's book *Awaken the Giant Within,* two friends were sick and tired of starting an exercise program or diet and never actually succeeding. So they made a public bet that if they wavered from their program, they would each have to eat a can of dog food. Whenever they were tempted to skip their workout or not follow their nutrition plan, they would go and read the can's ingredients label listing horse meat, etc., and their urges to get off track would quickly disappear.

Try to come up with a painful consequence to not following your program. In contrast, try to associate extreme pleasure with sticking to your plan and achieving your goals. You might reward yourself with a $1,000 shopping spree, a weeklong trip to a spa or a well-deserved day off or holiday. Go back to your notes and make sure you have come up with enough painful consequences and pleasurable sensations that you will be certain to stick to the plan.

The motivation and inspiration to stick to your program is within you. You just have to find the right reason – the reason that will make you so emotionally charged that you will take action, make the changes and stick to them regularly.

WE CANNOT
STAND STILL.
WE MUST GROW.
WE MUST KEEP
ON IMPROVING
OURSELF. THIS
IS LIFE'S MAIN
ISSUE. ALL THE
EXPERIENCES OF
LIFE ARE FOR
THE PURPOSE OF
MAKING US MORE
WONDERFUL.

ELINOR
MACDONALD

Here is an example to demonstrate this phenomenon. Imagine you are on the 28th floor of a high-rise building. There is a small two-by-four wooden plank that extends from the window of your building to the building on the opposite side of the street. In the other building, there is a man who is holding a $100 bill and will give it to you if you walk across the plank to the other side. You look down 28 storeys, you see the cars speeding by and your stomach turns into a knot. Would you go for $100? Probably not. Would you go for $1,000? Still no way. It is not worth it! But now imagine the man is threatening to shoot one of your closest loved ones – your spouse, daughter, son or grandchild – if you do not walk over. Now it is a different story. You would probably, without a doubt, without even thinking about it, walk the plank.

You can see by this dramatic example that the ability to walk the plank is always there. It is never a question of ability. You just need to find that strong reason to walk the plank – to do something you would really rather not do. Perhaps just losing 10 pounds or decreasing your risk for cardiovascular disease is like $100 – not enough reason to walk the plank or take action toward your goals. You will need to get more emotionally charged in order to stick to your plan. It's like brushing your teeth every morning. You would never consider not brushing your teeth. It's something you do without even thinking about it. It's non-negotiable. Discover what it is going to take for you, and remember, everyone is different. What is going to motivate me is not necessarily going to motivate you. Spend some time thinking about this, because motivation is what will establish the foundation for your success. Refer to your pain and pleasure lists regularly to help remind you why you have chosen to become healthier and fitter.

Step 3. YOUR GOALS MUST BE SMART.

The next series of homework assignments will help you move closer to achieving your fat loss goals by mapping out your particular route. For a nutrition and fitness program to succeed, it must be personalized. As with motivation, your goals will be your own.

In the following space, write down all the fitness goals you would like to achieve. It is your personal fitness wish list. Remember when you were a kid making up your Christmas wish list? You wrote down everything under the sun. You did not care whether you thought you would actually get it or not. You wrote it anyways. That is what I want you to do. I want you to write down anything you have ever thought of achieving with regards to your health and fitness. Which health and fitness goal, if you achieved it, would make this year unbelievable? Have you ever wanted to hike the Grand Canyon, complete a marathon, cycle through Italy or learn to scuba dive? Would you be happy just with working out four times a week consistently? What are your health and fitness wishes?

_____

_____

_____

_____

_____

_____

_____

_____

_____

_____

_____

_____

_____

Setting realistic goals is the key to success. But it is not enough to say, "I want to get into shape." Effective and realistic goals are Specific, Measurable, Attainable, Reward-based and have a Time frame. Here are some examples of SMART goals.

- *Hike the Grand Canyon for one week this May.*
- *Run on the treadmill for 10 minutes three times a week by November 3.*
- *Resistance train every Monday, Wednesday and Friday until December 31.*
- *Train for and complete the half marathon on September 10.*
- *Exercise on the cardio machines for one hour without stopping by February 1.*
- *Work out with a personal trainer two times a week for the next six months, then reassess.*
- *Sign up for the scuba diving course that starts March 1.*
- *Drink six glasses of water every day by June 1.*
- *Eat five small meals or snacks every day by March 1.*

Each goal is clear, easy to measure and has a deadline. You will notice that none of the goals I have listed include anything about body weight or size. Deciding to lose 10 pounds is an outcome-oriented goal. I prefer to use behaviour- or action-oriented goals. I firmly believe my approach is a lot more positive. For example, in the process of training for a half marathon, you will definitely lose body fat, but your focus is on something much more positive.

HOMEWORK

1. Go back to your fitness wish list and make sure each goal is Specific, Measurable, Attainable and has a Time frame. Revise all your goals to make them as SMART as possible and rewrite them in the following space. Avoid setting any weight or fat loss goals. Instead focus on the actions you can take that will promote fat loss.

_____

_____

_____

_____

_____

_____

_____

_____

_____

_____

_____

_____

_____

_____

2. But don't stop there. Successful goal setting requires two more things. Be prepared to reassess and reevaluate your goals on a regular basis and reward yourself once you have achieved a goal. For example, treat yourself to a massage, a new outfit or a trip. Then set your sights on the next goals. Go back to your goals and attach a reward to each one. Be sure that the reward is motivating enough to encourage you to stick to your plan.

3. Sometimes, when starting an exercise or nutrition program, we can get overzealous and decide to change a million things all at once. It soon becomes clear that we have taken on too much, and it becomes almost impossible to succeed at anything. To avoid this, you need to determine what is most important to you and focus on that first. Once you have got that under control, you can move on to your next goal. Go back to your list and number your goals in order of priority, with number one for the goal that is most important to you and which you would like to achieve first.

ITSY-BITSY BABY STEPS

If you are undertaking a major lifestyle change, the big picture may be a bit overwhelming. Take the big goal and split it into small, easily achievable goals. This is realistic. It will help you succeed on a regular basis, and that will give you the momentum you need to reach the ultimate goal.

HOMEWORK

Go back to your fitness wish list. Take the top three goals from your list and break them down into smaller goals that will act as milestones toward your ultimate goal. For example, if your number one goal is to complete a half marathon, here's how you'd break it down into smaller action steps.

1. Enroll in the local half-marathon running clinic.

2. Purchase new footwear and clothing.

3. Consult with a personal trainer for two sessions to get help with designing my program.

4. Schedule three morning runs a week with friends.

5. Register and pay for the local six-mile (10-km) fun run midway through my training program.

6. Register and pay for the half-marathon event.

ACTION STEPS:

Goal #1 =

ACTION STEP #1: _____

ACTION STEP #2: _____

ACTION STEP #3: _____

ACTION STEP #4: _____

ACTION STEP #5: _____

ACTION STEP #6: _____

Goal #2 =

ACTION STEP #1: _____

ACTION STEP #2: _____

ACTION STEP #3: _____

ACTION STEP #4: _____

ACTION STEP #5: _____

ACTION STEP #6: _____

Goal #3 = _____

ACTION STEP #1: _____

ACTION STEP #2: _____

ACTION STEP #3: _____

ACTION STEP #4: _____

ACTION STEP #5: _____

ACTION STEP #6: _____

> IF YOU MUST
> BEGIN THEN
> GO ALL THE WAY,
> BECAUSE IF YOU
> BEGIN AND QUIT,
> THE UNFINISHED
> BUSINESS YOU
> HAVE LEFT
> BEHIND BEGINS
> TO HAUNT YOU
> ALL THE
> TIME.
>
> CHOGYAM
> TRUNGPA

Step 4. OBSTACLES AND STRATEGIES

You have most likely tried to lose weight before. Most people have. They try over and over again. Something like a New Year's resolution, summer, a wedding or a reunion motivates them to try again. Each time they fail because they are basically mimicking exactly what they did the last time. They decide they will just stop eating breakfast and lunch or they will exercise for two hours every day. This represents a definition of insanity – doing the same thing over and over again but expecting a different result. Whatever forced them off track last time will more than likely do so again.

This time, things are going to be different. This time you are going to be prepared. We are going to develop a strategy for overcoming roadblocks posed by work, kids, fatigue or lack of time. We are going to determine how you are going to balance it all. For example, if previously you found work or family responsibilities got in the way of you achieving your goals, your strategy might be to book your workout appointments into your schedule as you would any other appointment. You would not cancel a business appointment with an important client or cancel your yearly physical with your doctor. Likewise, you must never cancel your workouts.

Another strategy might be to hire a personal trainer, which will force you to keep your exercise appointment, or ask a friend to join you in a commitment to walk every day at lunch. Perhaps you find that at about two months into your program, you always get bored with what you are doing and eventually give up. This time you could plan to consult with a personal trainer just before this happens, so you avoid getting off track. Or you could make a list of new activities you will try every two months.

Outline any obstacles that have surfaced in the past or that you expect will surface in the future. Once you have outlined the potential obstacles, you can determine your strategies for overcoming them. You will be prepared – no surprises!

OBSTACLES TO FITNESS

OBSTACLE	STRATEGY
	(you might find it necessary to outline numerous strategies for any potential obstacle)
1.	
2.	
3.	
4.	
5.	

> EACH
> PROBLEM
> HAS HIDDEN IN
> IT AN OPPORTUNITY
> SO POWERFUL
> THAT IT LITERALLY
> DWARFS THE
> PROBLEM. THE
> GREAT SUCCESS
> STORIES WERE
> CREATED BY
> PEOPLE WHO
> RECOGNIZED A
> PROBLEM AND
> TURNED IT
> INTO AN
> OPPORTUNITY.
>
> ANONYMOUS

Eighty percent of people still do not exercise consistently enough to enjoy any health benefits. Here are the most common stumbling blocks to exercise and healthy ways to overcome them.

I don't have enough time. If you have trouble finding time to exercise, you are not alone. A perceived lack of time is one of the most common excuses for not starting or for quitting an exercise program. But it really does not wash. I have clients who manage large businesses, clients with six to eight children and clients who seem to do it all. How do they do it? They make health and fitness a priority in their life. When life gets rough, exercise is usually the first thing to go when, in fact, it should be the last. Exercise is the key to mental sanity when life becomes chaotic.

Somehow, when others need you, your needs tend to end up on the back burner. Someone at work asks you to complete a project, your spouse needs your attention, the kids need some quality time, your friends are asking you why you have not called and you have a to-do list that extends well into the next six months. You can see how easy it is to convince yourself that the morning jog can wait until lunch and then until after dinner. Or maybe until tomorrow and, finally, you think, "I'll get back on track next month." Commitments, responsibilities and the demands of work, family and social life are always going to be there. When you allow yourself to put your own needs second to everything and everyone else, you will end up the loser.

Research shows that people who exercise are more productive at whatever they are doing. Translation: You will be able to do more when you are in good shape. As for believing exercise is a huge time commitment, even 10 to 30 minutes a day, if done consistently, can result in health benefits.

Make an appointment with yourself, just as you would with your doctor or dentist or for a meeting with your boss. That way, when someone asks if you can meet at 5:00, you can honestly say, "Sorry, I've got an appointment. How about at 4:00?" Scheduling fitness into your life is why personal trainers have become so popular. Now you are accountable to your trainer as well as yourself.

Stop putting it off! "I'll start exercising right after New Year's . . . in the spring . . . right after I'm finished with this huge project . . . once the kids get older . . . once the kids leave home . . . after I've retired . . ." Stop making excuses. Now is the time to start because there will always be things competing for your time. You can choose to make exercise a priority in your life now or wait until you're forced to make it a priority. Have you ever heard the saying "People who cannot find the time to exercise will one day be forced to find the time for illness"? We take our health for granted until we get sick. People who swear they do not have a minute to exercise, then find themselves hospitalized for heart bypass surgery and out of commission for weeks soon recognize that the extra time taken to exercise would haven been well worth it. The message is clear. Unless you take care of yourself now, one day you might find yourself unable to take care of your business, your family or any of your other interests.

Another helpful strategy for overcoming the time obstacle is to sit down and record how you spend your time in a typical day. Then go through the list and identify any time wasters. These could include the television or computer, or perhaps there is someone at work who constantly interrupts you, making you less efficient. Now determine how you could avoid some of these time wasters. For example, if someone at work takes up a portion of your time, make it known that from 10:00 until noon, you are not to be interrupted so you can focus on some important projects. I think you will find that you do have time to exercise. You just need to restructure your schedule to make sure you have time for the most important person in your life – yourself.

I have no energy. Those who exercise regularly know from experience that exercise actually leaves you with more energy. Some helpful strategies for overcoming this obstacle are to schedule exercise when you are less likely to feel exhausted from a long day at work or with the kids. Get up 45 minutes earlier than everyone else and go for a walk. This will start your day off on a positive note. Keep your fitness gear in the car so that on the way home you can stop at the gym for your workout. If you go home first, the couch and TV might be too tempting after a long day at work. Or, if you do find yourself skipping out on your workouts because you have no energy, schedule your workouts with a trainer or a friend. Whether you are tired or not, you still have to be there, because they are waiting for you.

I'm too old to start exercising. No, you are too old **not** to exercise! With every passing decade, a 30-year-old sedentary individual will experience a 10 percent decrease in muscle mass and aerobic capacity and a reduction in flexibility. Bone density deteriorates starting at age 35. By the time you are 68, you will have experienced an 80 percent decrease in strength. By age 80, an individual will have lost half of their muscle mass. The good news is that if you exercise, these statistics will improve dramatically. Even people as old as 90 have experienced the positive benefits of exercise, so it is never too late to get started. The American Surgeon General's Report indicates that 30 minutes of activity every day is enough to achieve various health benefits. The level of activity is equivalent to gardening, performing household chores or light walking or cycling. Consider enrolling in a line-dancing or ballroom-dancing program. Perhaps tai chi or yoga is enticing. The exercise does not have to be intense, but you do need to start doing something.

> OBSTACLES ARE A NATURAL PART OF LIFE, JUST AS BOULDERS ARE A NATURAL PART OF THE COURSE OF THE RIVER. THE RIVER DOES NOT COMPLAIN OR GET DEPRESSED BECAUSE THERE ARE BOULDERS IN ITS PATH.
>
> I CHING

> CONTINUOUS EFFORT – NOT STRENGTH OR INTELLIGENCE – IS THE KEY TO UNLOCKING OUR POTENTIAL.
>
> LIANE CORDES

I hate exercise. In the beginning, exercise might feel like a chore, but eventually it will become a physical and mental-health need. It is important to find activities you enjoy doing so that you will participate in them regularly, see the results and get hooked. Use music, try hiking or walking, and add variety to your program to make it more fun. Exercise with friends. Studies show people tend to achieve better results that way, because it becomes more difficult to skip workouts.

There is also no evidence to suggest that exercise needs to be painful. If it hurts that much, you might be doing too much too soon. While exercising, you might feel some discomfort, muscular fatigue or a burning sensation near the end of a set or an exercise bout. These feelings are normal. However, while performing an exercise, you should not feel sharp pain. This is not normal, and you should stop the exercise immediately and consult a sports physician or physiotherapist.

All of us have experienced muscle soreness after a new activity or highly intense workout. Remember the feeling after your first day of skiing, first aerobics class or the first run of the summer? This sensation is referred to as delayed-onset muscle soreness, because it usually kicks in one to three days after the workout. Many participants rate the effectiveness of a workout by how sore they are afterwards. But if you are training appropriately, there is no need to be sore. It is okay to think, "Hey, my muscles feel like they had a great workout yesterday." However, if you have a problem getting out of a chair, walking or even just moving, you are training too hard – and not very sensibly.

To reduce the likelihood of extreme muscle soreness from training sessions, always warm up, cool down, stretch and progress slowly. Once you have established a consistent exercise routine, there are no extra health benefits from pushing yourself to be extremely sore. Remember, pain is a warning signal that your body has done too much too soon. When you experience extreme muscle soreness or pain, back off on the intensity of your program and progress more slowly. "No pain, no gain" is a myth. Pain is not necessary to improve your fitness and get results.

I'm too out of shape to exercise. One survey found that the top reason why people choose not to join a gym is because they want to get into better shape or lose weight first. This backwards approach might never get you to your goals. Find a gym that is not intimidating and where members seem comfortable going at their own pace and wearing whatever they want, or work out in the privacy of your own home or neighbourhood.

The gym scene is not my thing. Sorry, this will not fly. There are literally hundreds of things you can do at home to get in shape. Your local bookstore will have books on designing your own program. Rent a fitness video. Hire a personal trainer to come to your house and design a program for you.

My knees hurt, so I can't exercise. The health benefits of exercise often outweigh the risks. Certain conditions might make exercise more difficult, but you can work around most problems. Consult with a professional who can design a program that addresses your specific concerns. For example, if you do have knee problems, there is no reason why you cannot work on your upper body and abdominals while you rehabilitate your knees.

I can't see any results. One of the biggest hurdles new exercisers face is that the effort often does not match the result. They have been exercising religiously for five weeks and jump on the scale. Ugh, no change! They feel the program must not be working and give up. Unrealistic expectations can be a real downer. Instead of measuring your success by the scale, measure it by your energy levels. Monitor how many more repetitions you can do of a particular exercise. Keep track of how many more minutes you can spend doing a given activity. You may be making more progress than you think. (See chapter 2 for more suggestions on monitoring your success.)

PERSISTENCE COUNTS

Sticking to an exercise or nutrition program takes a lot of discipline. Sometimes wanting to do the right thing can slip us up if we have the wrong attitude about it. Do you see yourself in any of the following scenarios?

ALL OR NOTHING

You are scheduled for a 90-minute workout, but something comes up and you cannot get to the gym for the allocated time. You scrap the workout and decide you will try to fit it in tomorrow. You have decided to eat healthier, but one day you slip a bit at lunch and have a chocolate bar. You decide that since you have already failed for the day, you might as well throw in the towel and indulge in a few cookies, a bowl of ice cream and a bag of chips. Tomorrow is another day. Can you see how this "all or nothing" approach works against you? Wouldn't a 30-minute workout have been better than no exercise as all? Wouldn't a single chocolate bar have been better than an all-out binge? Sometimes striving for perfection is what leads to failure. The trick in trying to stick to a long-term plan is to learn to compromise. When it comes to nutrition, for example, focus on the 80/20 rule – 80 percent of the time you eat really well and 20 percent of the time you indulge a little. No going overboard, though. When it comes to exercise, remember that any activity is better than nothing.

THE MORE I CAN LOVE EVERYTHING – THE TREES, THE LAND, THE WATER, MY FELLOW MEN, WOMEN AND CHILDREN, AND MYSELF – THE MORE HEALTH I AM GOING TO EXPERIENCE AND THE MORE OF MYSELF I AM GOING TO BE.

CARL SIMONTON

WHEN WE GET
INTO A TIGHT
PLACE AND
EVERYTHING GOES
AGAINST YOU
TILL IT SEEMS AS
THOUGH YOU
COULD NOT
HOLD ON FOR
ONE MINUTE
LONGER, NEVER
GIVE UP THEN,
FOR THAT IS
JUST THE PLACE
THAT THE TIDE
WILL TURN.

HARRIET
BEECHER
STOWE

So many of us fall prey to the lure of immediate gratification. The chocolate cake staring us in the face is too great a temptation compared to future weight loss. We would rather experience the pleasure now and worry about the consequences later. A binge today simply means tomorrow we will eat better or we will work out twice as long or hard. There is always a way to justify a lack of discipline. Discipline and willpower are perceived as deprivation – we are sacrificing or losing something. But try to remember that each time you work out, stick to a nutritional plan or decide not to indulge in a less-healthy choice, you are actually giving yourself something – spiritually, emotionally and physically.

Sticking to an exercise or nutrition plan is the same as practising self-discipline when your kids are driving you nuts. You would like to scream, shout and lose it, but instead you count to 10 and choose your words carefully. There is no doubt that practicing this type of discipline makes you feel better about yourself. It is the same with exercise. Your body deserves to be treated well. You deserve to eat well and exercise regularly. Many athletes think of their body as a temple, and so should you. Think of this the next time you notice yourself reaching for another piece of cake. Push it away and consider that you are actually giving yourself something rather than taking something away.

HOMEWORK

1. List ways you have been known to sometimes sabotage your efforts.

----

2. List ways you will commit to changing your approach so your behaviours will support your efforts.

_____

_____

_____

_____

_____

_____

_____

_____

_____

_____

_____

_____

_____

_____

_____

_____

You should be very proud of yourself! By taking the time to answer all of the questions in this section, you have set up a framework for success. It is so much easier to get to your destination if you have a map.

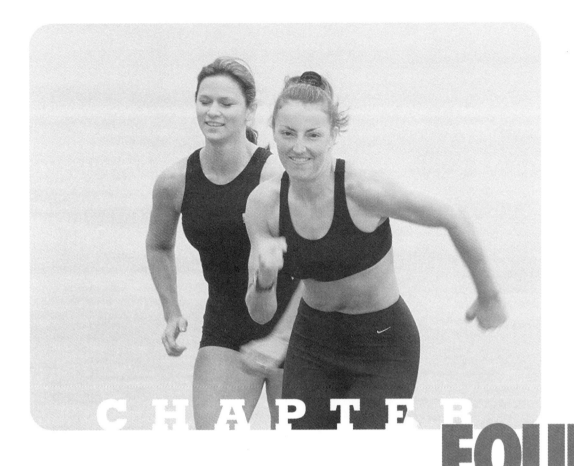

CHAPTER

FOUR

DESIGNING YOUR FAT LOSS EXERCISE PROGRAM

CARDIOVASCULAR

EXERCISE

This aspect of your program will be critical. During this stage you will be burning fat directly and getting closer to your fat loss goals.

The American College of Sports Medicine (ACSM) recommends five to seven days per week of cardiovascular aerobic activity to maximize fat loss. It is suggested that each aerobic session expend 300 calories minimum to be categorized as a fat loss workout. This would be equivalent to approximately 32 minutes of stepping or a high-intensity fitness class, three miles (4.8 km) of running or five miles (8 km) of walking. The actual type of aerobic activity must be continuous in nature and involve your large muscle groups. Some of the best choices are as follows.

- *walking*
- *running*
- *cycling*
- *swimming*
- *in-line skating*
- *hiking*

- *rowing*
- *racquet sports*
- *cross-country skiing*
- *stair climbing*
- *fitness classes*

A HORSE
THAT RESISTS
THE REINS, A
CAR WITHOUT
BRAKES AND A
PERSON WITH
NO SELF-CONTROL
ARE ALL EQUALLY
HEADED FOR
DISASTER.

SATHYA
SAI BABA

CHOOSING AN AEROBIC ACTIVITY

The most important consideration when deciding upon your primary fat loss activity is deciding which of the listed activities interests you the most and that you really believe you could adhere to on an ongoing basis. The best fat loss aerobic activity in the world is the one you actually do regularly. If I told you that running was the best way to burn fat but you hated running, you probably would not stick to the program very well and, of course, would experience very limited results. So you really need to examine your interests. For example, if you prefer to exercise outside, running along trails or hiking might be your answer. If you prefer to exercise indoors, you might enjoy the energy of fitness classes or running on a treadmill so you can be distracted by a magazine or TV. If you like to exercise in a group, fitness classes or a running clinic might help you stick to your program. If you are a solo exerciser, your own individualized program might offer the solitude you are looking for. A good personal trainer will ask her clients a number of questions before developing an exercise program. It is important to determine the perfect-fit, custom-designed program that will facilitate your efforts.

HOMEWORK

Answer the following questions to help you determine which activities you would be best suited for.

How many days per week can your schedule accommodate exercise? _____

How much time do you want to commit during each exercise session? _____

Which days are best for you to exercise?   M   T   W   T   F   S   S

Which days are best for you to rest?   M   T   W   T   F   S   S

Do you like to exercise in the morning, at midday or in the evening? _____

Do you like to exercise alone, with a friend, in a group or a combination? _____

What kind of exercise is most appealing or interesting to you? Why?

_____

_____

_____

_____

_____

PUTTING YOU THROUGH YOUR PACES

Part of a personal trainer's job is to prescribe a type of exercise that is going to be easy for their client to do. In order to find out what this might be, a trainer needs to ask a few important questions about a person's likes and dislikes. You do not need a personal trainer to help you find out for yourself what exercise choices might be appropriate for you. For example, if you like exercising alone, enrolling in a group fitness class might set you up for failure. Or if you hate running, starting a running program might not be the best idea. PACES, or the Physical ACtivity Enjoyment Scale, is a great way to gauge whether your choice of activity is the best one for you.

PACES works like this. Let's say you want to become more active and are looking for a sport that meets a number of your needs, including cardiovascular training, greater muscle strength and endurance, and the chance to enlarge your social circle. Your friend has suggested you try volleyball. You would use the following PACES chart to determine if the activity is right for you. Circle the number that best applies to you and the activity you are considering. Add up your total score. If your score is less than 30, you experience extreme enjoyment from the activity. This would suggest that your choice is probably the right one for you. If you score is between 30 and 50, you might benefit from varying the exercise or trying something different. If your score is greater than 50, you are probably doing the wrong exercise and should try something else.

Remember that consistency is the primary key to achieving your exercise goals. Find an activity you enjoy and you will be more motivated to participate, stick with it and reap the benefits more quickly. Find which activity sparks your interest, and soon you will also enjoy a fit and healthier body.

HOMEWORK

Complete the following chart for three separate activities and refer to the above notes to analyze your scores.

MEN OFTEN BECOME WHAT THEY BELIEVE THEMSELVES TO BE. IF I BELIEVE I CANNOT DO SOMETHING, IT MAKES ME INCAPABLE OF DOING IT. BUT WHEN I BELIEVE I CAN, THEN I ACQUIRE THE ABILITY TO DO IT EVEN IF I DIDN'T HAVE IT IN THE BEGINNING.

MOHANDAS GANDHI

PACES (PHYSICAL ACTIVITY ENJOYMENT SCALE)

ACTIVITY: _____

	1	2	3	4	5	
I find it pleasurable.						I find it unpleasant.
I feel interested.						I feel bored.
I like it.						I dislike it.
I am very absorbed in this activity.						I am not at all absorbed.
It is a lot of fun.						It is no fun at all.
I find it energizing.						I find it tiring.
It makes me happy.						It makes me depressed.
It is very pleasant.						It is very unpleasant.
I feel good doing it.						I feel bad doing it.
It is very invigorating.						It is not invigorating.
I am not at all frustrated by it.						I am frustrated by it.
It is very gratifying.						It is not at all gratifying.
It is very exhilarating.						It is not at all exhilarating.
It is very stimulating.						It is not at all stimulating.
It gives me a strong sense of accomplishment.						It does not give me a sense of accomplishment.
It is very refreshing.						It is not at all refreshing.
I feel as though there is nothing else I would rather be doing.						I feel as though I would rather be doing something else.
I enjoy it.						I hate it.

TOTAL: _____

PACES (PHYSICAL ACTIVITY ENJOYMENT SCALE)

ACTIVITY: _____

	1	2	3	4	5	
I find it pleasurable.						I find it unpleasant.
I feel interested.						I feel bored.
I like it.						I dislike it.
I am very absorbed in this activity.						I am not at all absorbed.
It is a lot of fun.						It is no fun at all.
I find it energizing.						I find it tiring.
It makes me happy.						It makes me depressed.
It is very pleasant.						It is very unpleasant.
I feel good doing it.						I feel bad doing it.
It is very invigorating.						It is not invigorating.
I am not at all frustrated by it.						I am frustrated by it.
It is very gratifying.						It is not at all gratifying.
It is very exhilarating.						It is not at all exhilarating.
It is very stimulating.						It is not at all stimulating.
It gives me a strong sense of accomplishment.						It does not give me a sense of accomplishment.
It is very refreshing.						It is not at all refreshing.
I feel as though there is nothing else I would rather be doing.						I feel as though I would rather be doing something else.
I enjoy it.						I hate it.

TOTAL: _____

PACES (PHYSICAL ACTIVITY ENROYMENT SCALE)

PACES (PHYSICAL ACTIVITY ENJOYMENT SCALE)

ACTIVITY: _____

	1	2	3	4	5	
I find it pleasurable.						I find it unpleasant.
I feel interested.						I feel bored.
I like it.						I dislike it.
I am very absorbed in this activity.						I am not at all absorbed.
It is a lot of fun.						It is no fun at all.
I find it energizing.						I find it tiring.
It makes me happy.						It makes me depressed.
It is very pleasant.						It is very unpleasant.
I feel good doing it.						I feel bad doing it.
It is very invigorating.						It is not invigorating.
I am not at all frustrated by it.						I am frustrated by it.
It is very gratifying.						It is not at all gratifying.
It is very exhilarating.						It is not at all exhilarating.
It is very stimulating.						It is not at all stimulating.
It gives me a strong sense of accomplishment.						It does not give me a sense of accomplishment.
It is very refreshing.						It is not at all refreshing.
I feel as though there is nothing else I would rather be doing.						I feel as though I would rather be doing something else.
I enjoy it.						I hate it.

TOTAL: _____

Do not skip the PACES charts. Too many people start a running program when they actually hate running, sign up for an aerobics class when they actually like working out by themselves or decide to train on Fridays when Fridays are normally hectic for them.

Record your top three preferred aerobic activities, based on their PACES scores.

1. _____

2. _____

3. _____

Based on all your answers in this section, you can now develop a daily exercise program you will want to stick with.

HOMEWORK

Design your own personalized cardiovascular exercise program using the chart below.

Do not worry about "making mistakes" in your program. Just getting you to exercise regularly is all we need to do at this point. You can fine-tune your program as you go along and as I introduce you to some fat loss-maximizing concepts. For now, just remember that the best fat loss program in the world is the one you do regularly. So just get moving and never stop!

PERSONAL EXERCISE PROGRAM

ACTIVITY	MON.	TUES.	WED.	THURS.	FRI.	SAT.	SUN.

> EVERY MAN
> IS THE BUILDER
> OF THE TEMPLE
> CALLED HIS
> BODY — WE ARE
> ALL SCULPTORS
> AND PAINTERS,
> AND OUR
> MATERIAL IS
> OUR FLESH AND
> BLOOD AND
> BONES. ANY
> NOBLENESS BEGINS
> AT ONCE TO
> REFINE A MAN'S
> FEATURES.
>
> HENRY DAVID
> THOREAU

Review your program. Does it look realistic? Most people who start an exercise program are initially very excited, motivated and ready to commit to anything. Unfortunately, this enthusiasm might not last long if the goals they have set are unrealistic.

If you have never exercised consistently before, do not make any dramatic changes in your lifestyle. Although you might believe you can commit to working out five times a week, for example, you might find it difficult to keep this up. It is better to set smaller goals in the beginning. Attempt to exercise two days a week for a month, and if you succeed – excellent – advance your program. If you set a goal to exercise five times each week and miss a number of workouts, you will feel like a failure even if you worked out four times that week. Achieving small goals gives you the momentum to achieve the next set of goals.

Setting small, more manageable goals introduces exercise into your lifestyle gradually and, since you are still doing a lot more than you were doing before, you are going to see results. After a month or two, increase your weekly exercise frequency slowly and gradually. With my clients, I make small changes to their exercise routines every six to eight weeks in order to keep the program fresh, exciting and different.

Wait about six months before graduating to high-intensity exercise if you are a beginner. You do not want to start by dreading each exercise session because you know it is going to hurt. That will make it difficult to stay motivated. Three easy walks a week on an ongoing basis is far better than one hard run every once in a while. Remember, consistency is the key to getting results. You are going to eventually want to intensify your program and make a good effort at each workout, but you should progress to this level slowly.

FINE-TUNING YOUR FAT LOSS EXERCISE PROGRAM

Before we move on, I would like you to examine the following considerations. We know that in order to maximize caloric expenditure, we need to maximize the amount of oxygen we are consuming. We utilize more oxygen when we involve more muscle mass. So any activities that involve more muscle mass will make your fat loss program a lot more efficient. Consider these points.

- At least one or two of your primary aerobic activities should involve activities during which you stand to perform them, such as running, power walking, cross-country skiing or stair climbing. If your muscles have to support you in an upright position, they must expend more energy than if you were seated, with your body weight supported.

- At least one of your primary aerobic activities should involve both your arms and your legs. Activities such as rowing and cross-country skiing, which involve vigorous activity by both your arms and your legs, will expend a lot of energy. For example cross-country skiing, which occurs in an upright position and involves both your arms and your legs, burns more calories than rowing.

- The environment in which you exercise may affect fat loss. Your heat regulator and your appetite are both controlled by your hypothalamus. So, if you are exercising in a cold-er environment, like a pool during a swim workout, your hypothalamus must act in order to maintain your core temperature. As it responds to the colder environment, it also acts to stimulate your appetite. This explains why many athletes find they might start a run hungry but once they are finished, they might not be ready to eat for an hour or more. This effect is even greater if the run took place on a hot day. In contrast, many athletes have difficulty explaining why, after a swim workout or a long, easy hike, they are famished. This effect makes it more difficult to lose fat with swimming. This is why elite-level swimmers still carry on average five percent more body fat than elite-level runners. I am definitely not suggesting that you find the hottest environment in which to perform your workouts – which would pose its own health risks. I am also not suggesting that swimming does not burn fat. It is just not as efficient as, say, running. Swimming has many advantages for overweight individuals. Their bodies do not overheat, so the workout feels more comfortable; the buoyancy factor makes the exercise a lot easier on the joints; and they can definitely improve their cardiovascular and musculoskeletal systems. Just be sure that not all your primary workouts consist of activities like swimming, outdoor cycling and easy hiking, which all take place in a colder environment. Instead, include at least one activity during which you will sweat and raise your body's core temperature.

> IN ALL HUMAN AFFAIRS THERE ARE EFFORTS, AND THERE ARE RESULTS, AND THE STRENGTH OF THE EFFORT IS THE MEASURE OF THE RESULT. CHANCE IS NOT.
>
> JAMES ALLEN

HOMEWORK

Review your Personal Exercise Program and make any necessary adjustments based on what you learned in the previous section.

> THE BODY IS
> THE SOUL'S
> HOUSE.
> SHOULDN'T
> WE TAKE
> CARE OF OUR
> HOUSE SO
> THAT IT
> DOESN'T
> FALL INTO
> RUIN?
>
> PHILO

You might remember that a few years ago, many fitness professionals were prescribing lower intensity activity to maximize fat loss. Many fit people lowered the intensity of their workouts, fearful that they were not burning fat. Unfortunately, they were misled, and many people still believe that low-intensity activity is the best way to maximize fat loss. The reality is that the activity that expends the greatest number of calories will lead to the greatest amount of fat burned.

Yes, during lower intensity activity you will burn a higher percentage of fat and during higher intensity activity you will burn a higher percentage of carbohydrates or sugars. But the important point to note is that during low-intensity activity, you are burning fat at a higher percentage of a **lower number of calories**. When you exercise at a lower intensity, you are definitely expending fewer calories. The selective use of fat as a fuel, specifically at lower intensities, does not translate into greater fat loss, regardless of how tempting it is to draw this conclusion. The more important focus with regard to calories expended is not the percentage of energy coming from fat, but rather the total volume of fat used and the total number of calories expended. Let me show you the math. For our purposes, a kilocalorie (kcal) is the same as a calorie.

At 60% of maximum heart rate (easier intensity):

- *approximately 50% of calories come from fat (50% from sugars)*
- *approximately 8 kcal/min. are expended*
- *60 minutes x 8 kcal/min. = 480 total kilocalories*
- *50% x 480 kcal = 240 fat calories*

At 80% of maximum heart rate (more vigorous intensity):

- *approximately 40% of calories come from fat (60% from sugars)*
- *approximately 11 kcal/min. are expended*
- *60 minutes x 11 kcal/min. = 640 total calories*
- *40% x 640 kcal = 264 fat calories*

From these figures you can see how fitness leaders could have been misled. If you were to examine only the first line, the percentage of fat being burned as fuel, you would definitely prescribe lower intensity activity. However, if you examine the whole picture, it is clear that higher intensity activity definitely expends more calories and also more fat. Here are some more statistics to convince you.

It takes approximately 3,500 calories to burn one pound (0.45 kg) of fat. Compare the following exercise programs.

Program A
Easier intensity (approximately 5 kcal/min.), for example, easy walking

- *30 minutes of activity three times per week*
- *150 kcal/session x 3/week = 450 kcal/week*
- *3,500 kcal ÷ 450 kcal/week = 7.7 weeks*
- *It would take about 8 weeks to burn one pound (0.45 kg) of fat.*

Program B
Same intensity as above but for a longer duration

- *60 minutes of activity three times per week*
- *300 kcal/session x 3/week = 900 kcal/week*
- *3,500 kcal ÷ 900 kcal/week = 3.8 weeks*
- *It would take about four weeks to burn one pound (0.45 kg) of fat.*

Program C
More vigorous intensity (approximately 10 kcal/min.) , for example, jogging or power walking up and down hills

- *60 minutes of activity 3 times per week*
- *600 kcal/session x 3/week = 1,800 kcal/week*
- *3,500 kcal ÷ 1,800 kcal/week = 1.9 weeks*
- *It would take about two weeks to burn one pound (0.45 kg) of fat.*

> THE RIPPLE EFFECT DESCRIBES HOW A MINOR CHANGE IN BEHAVIOUR OR ATTITUDE CAN HAVE A MAJOR EFFECT.
>
> JOYCE BROTHERS

If you followed program A, it would take you eight weeks to burn one pound of fat. Most people would give up by then! If you could easily handle the higher intensity of program C, wouldn't you prefer to wait just two weeks to burn off that pound of fat deposited around your waist, hips or thighs? Remember, though, if you can't handle the higher intensity of program C, you could follow program B, which means you could maintain the easier intensity but would just have to work out for longer periods.

Time is definitely an issue for a lot of exercisers, and most don't want to spend hours in the gym if they can get the same results in a shorter period of time. Consider this: At 60 percent of your maximum heart rate, it would take you approximately 40 minutes to burn off 300 kcal. If you could handle a higher intensity and were able to exercise at 80 percent of your maximum heart rate, it would take you only approximately 27 minutes to burn the same 300 kcal. If time is a factor and you do not have a lot of time to waste, would you rather exercise for 40 or 27 minutes and still burn the same amount of calories?

YOU CAN BE
HEALED [OF
DEPRESSION]
IF EVERY DAY
YOU BEGIN
THE FIRST
THING IN THE
MORNING TO
CONSIDER HOW
YOU WILL BRING
A REAL JOY
TO SOMEONE
ELSE.

ALFRED
ADLER

Or what if you only had 36 minutes to work out? If you ran at an easy, 12-minute mile (0.13 km/min.) pace, you would expend approximately 298 kcal in that time period. But if you were able to sustain a more challenging, six-minute-mile pace (0.26 km/min.), you would expend 595 kcal in the same amount of time – double the expenditure.

If I have not convinced you yet, consider this. Did you know that the highest percentage of fat that you burn during any activity is during rest?! At rest, you are using approximately 50 percent fat as your fuel. (That is the highest percentage of fat you can burn; you are never burning 100 percent fat.) That's right, just sitting here reading this book, you are burning the highest percentage of fat you could possibly burn. That is because your body can only store a limited supply of carbohydrates (sugars) and so during rest, the demand on your body is low and your body wants to spare your precious sugar stores. Since you have an unlimited supply of fat stores, your body would rather burn fat during rest. But remember that although you are burning a higher percentage of fat at rest, you are expending very few calories (approximately 1 kcal/min.), so overall you are not burning a lot of fat. If type of fuel utilized were the critical factor for fat loss, then I would be prescribing more rest, because this is when we burn the highest percentage of fat as fuel. But it is a higher percentage of a **lower number of calories.** So, of course, we know it is ridiculous to even consider rest or sleep as a high-fat-burning activity.

One last note. Examine sprinters. The majority of their training sessions involve high-intensity, sugar-burning activity. But have you ever seen a fat sprinter? Of course not. Although they are burning a lot of carbohydrates or sugars during their training sessions, they are also expending a lot of calories and a lot of fat. In fact, sprinters can consume more than 5,000 kcal per day without gaining any fat!

The bottom line is that if you want to maximize fat loss, you need to maximize the number of calories you expend. An exercise physiologist's rule for fat loss is "Go as hard as you can, as long as you can, as often as you can." This type of prescription will definitely maximize fat loss; however, we do need to consider some other variables.

If you followed the prescription above, each training session might be so difficult that you would dread each of your workouts and might have a difficult time adhering to your program. You might find yourself skipping workouts, which would get you nowhere. In addition, if you followed this prescription, you might also start to experience numerous injuries or illnesses, because our bodies are not capable of going hard all the time. Instead, the recommended fat loss prescription is one that includes all intensity training zones. That is, sometimes you go easy for a longer period, and other times you go hard for a shorter period.

The best way to incorporate high-intensity exercise into your workouts is to include interval training, alternating between high-intensity bouts of exercise and low-intensity recovery periods. Use the following guidelines when designing your cardiovascular fat loss program.

YOUR WEEKLY AEROBIC PROGRAM

1. Schedule one to two short and intense interval workouts into your program each week. These workouts should last for approximately 20 minutes and should involve a rating of perceived exertion (RPE) intensity of approximately 8. (See the discussion of RPE at the end of this chapter.) During these workouts you will notice that your breathing is heavier and you will definitely be able to feel your heart beating more quickly. These workouts will definitely be above your comfort zone or where you would prefer to exercise. The benefits of this type of workout are as follows.

- *You expend more calories per minute.*

- *It's more efficient – you burn more calories in less time.*

- *It's an effective method for improving fitness conditioning*

- *It's effective at raising your anaerobic threshold. Your anaerobic threshold is the stage of exercise where you feel very tired and feel the need to either stop or slow down. You may experience dizziness or nausea if you stay at this level too long. By incorporating higher intensity activity into your exercise, you raise your anaerobic threshold. This means that you can exercise at a higher intensity before you start to experience those uncomfortable sensations.*

- *It's an effective method for inducing training adaptations. Incorporating this type of training into your program will enable your body to handle the higher intensities more easily. You will find that intensities that used to leave you breathless and fatigued no longer challenge you. Soon you will be able to expend more calories per minute compared to when you first started to exercise. When people initiate an exercise program, a comfortable calorie-burning level is approximately 5 cal/min. Elite athletes can expend more than 20 cal/min. and sustain this level for more than two hours. It obviously takes them a lot less time to burn one pound of fat.*

- *It's an effective method for increasing fat mobilization. This means that as you get fitter, you actually get better at burning fat. Inside your fat cells are enzymes called hormone-sensitive lipase and lipoprotein lipase. Hormone-sensitive lipase, the "good guys," are responsible for releasing fat from a fall cell to be used for energy. Lipoprotein lipase, the "bad guys," are responsible for the uptake of fat from the bloodstream to be stored in fat cells. Lipoprotein lipase functions to develop our unwanted bulges. If you have lived a*

ABOUT 90 PERCENT OF THE THINGS IN OUR LIVES ARE RIGHT AND ABOUT 10 PERCENT ARE WRONG. IF WE WANT TO BE HAPPY, ALL WE HAVE TO DO IS TO CONCENTRATE ON THE 90 PERCENT THAT ARE RIGHT AND IGNORE THE 10 PERCENT THAT ARE WRONG.

DALE CARNEGIE

THE GREATEST
IRRITANT TO
MOST PEOPLE
IS NOT THE
LACK OF MONEY
OR STATUS,
BUT ILL HEALTH.
NOTHING
SHINES BRIGHTLY
IF WE DO
NOT FEEL
WELL.

MARGARET
STORTZ

sedentary lifestyle and have eaten a poor diet all your life, you will have a lot of the bad guys, and they will be very good at their job. You will have fewer good guys, and they will not be so competent with their responsibilities. The goal is to get more good guys doing their job.

Changing the internal chemistry of your fat cells may take years. In the beginning you might not be experiencing results as quickly as you want because your body is actually working against you. But with consistency in your training program, your body will soon start to work for you. This is evident is someone who struggles with fat loss for months but maintains their commitment to their program. Eventually they express that they have not changed a thing but now it seems that the fat is falling off them. Finally they have increased their ability to mobilize and use fat as a fuel. Training in a high-intensity zone will increase your fitness level more quickly and enable you to enjoy this wonderful training benefit. Soon you will be burning more fat during and after exercise. You will become a fat-burning machine!

- *You experience a higher excess post oxygen consumption (EPOC). Have you ever wondered why you continue to breathe heavily after your workout is over? Why doesn't your breathing go back to normal immediately? After exercise you consume a greater amount of oxygen to assist your body in recovering from the stress of the workout and the demands it placed on your body. It is important to know that EPOC uses fat as its fuel. After higher intensity workouts, your EPOC is greater, translating into a greater caloric and fat expenditure post-activity. Although the effects of EPOC are small, if you expended an additional 100 calories postexercise as a result of a high-intensity exercise session, within 100 workouts you would have burned an extra 10,000 calories or three pounds (1.4 kg) of fat!*

- *The active recovery phases of interval training help avoid fatigue and injury.*

One important note: unfit individuals should not engage in high-intensity activity because of the potential danger. If you are just starting out, many of these tips will be inappropriate for you in the first few months. Of course, the faster you walk, step, dance, cycle or run, the more calories you use per minute. However, if you have been sedentary, high-intensity exercise compromises your ability to sustain exercise for a long time — and hence burn enough calories. For that reason, lower intensity exercise is more effective in the initial stages of training and is a prerequisite for higher intensity exercise that burns more calories. You will experience great results by just getting started on a program and will not need to implement any of these fine-tuning tips yet. If you did, you might risk injury and you might find it very difficult to adhere to your program.

Start by incorporating two months of easy training with a slow, gradual increase in volume. Do not worry about intensity. Just work on increasing the amount of time you spend exercising. You might initially schedule only two cardio sessions per week for one to two months, then progress from there, incorporating another day per week until you reach the ACSM recommendations for fat loss outlined at the beginning of this chapter.

2. Schedule one to two aerobic workouts of moderate length and intensity each week. These sessions should be 30 to 40 minutes long at an RPE level of 6 to 7. This is the intensity zone where most people will train, so this will feel comfortable. Most people neglect training in the extreme zones – the very easy and the very challenging.

3. Schedule two to three long, low-intensity workouts each week. These sessions should be at least 45 minutes long at an RPE intensity of 5. These workouts will definitely feel very comfortable. You might even feel as if you are going too slow. (You are not!) Workouts in this zone are not very stressful to your system but will effectively challenge and overload your aerobic-energy system and help to develop fat-burning enzymes. This intensity zone is also recommended if you are just beginning to exercise. The other zones may be too stressful and uncomfortable for you at this point.

HOMEWORK

Review your Personal Exercise Program you designed earlier and make any necessary adjustments in the following chart. Examine each workout and determine which workouts will be easy and long, which will be moderate in intensity and duration, and which will be hard but short.

> LEARN TO THRILL YOURSELF. . . . MAKE EVERYTHING BRIGHT AND BEAUTIFUL ABOUT YOU. CULTIVATE A SPIRIT OF HUMOUR. ENJOY THE SUNSHINE.
>
> **BAIRD SPALDING**

PERSONAL EXERCISE PROGRAM

ACTIVITY	MON.	TUES.	WED.	THURS.	FRI.	SAT.	SUN.

Here are some other helpful tips for you intermediate/advanced exerciser when designing your cardiovascular fat-burning program.

Include a six- to 12-minute low-intensity warm-up and cool-down. The body does not respond very well going from inactivity to very intense activity. The cardiovascular, musculoskeletal, neurological and metabolic energy pathways need to be gradually stimulated in order to perform at an optimal level. Muscles that are warm are more able to extract and utilize oxygen to produce energy. As muscles warm up, the enzyme activity level is increased. This means that fats and sugars are broken down more rapidly, and more energy and less lactic acid (the burning sensation) will be produced. This will enhance your performance and increase your ability to burn fat.

The body also does not respond very well going from intense activity to complete rest. Your heart, lungs, muscles, joints and energy systems require a gradual cool-down to avoid blood pooling in the lower extremities, to counteract dizziness and to assist in the recovery process. Warming up and cooling down is a healthy way to exercise anyways, but in addition, it is a way to prolong your caloric expenditure for each workout. So, for example, if you are going to go for a run, start and finish with a six-minute walk. A warm-up and cool-down should generally involve the same workout activity but at a much lower intensity.

Try a "cardio-split" program once or twice a week. In the morning when you wake up, go for a workout. You have been sleeping all night and your metabolism is low, so a workout is a great way to jump-start it and get you burning more calories right from the get-go. Then, as you go through your day, your metabolic rate remains relatively high. As you start to wind down and your metabolism is about to drop, go for an evening workout at approximately 6:00 to 8:00 p.m. The theory is that by "splitting" your cardio workouts you will maximize your metabolic rate and burn more calories in a 24-hour period. Try, for example, a walk in the morning and a fitness class in the evening.

Try an early-morning workout. When deciding when to exercise, consider that working out first thing in the morning has many advantages. One theory is that an early-morning workout will jump-start your metabolism and get you revving at a higher level all day long. In addition, and probably more importantly, many people find if they work out first thing and get it out of the way, there are less chances for life's responsibilities to distract them from their exercise ambitions. And, finally, an early-morning workout sets the tone for the entire day. You already have one success under your belt and thus may find it easier to make healthier choices at lunch or pass on the doughnut break mid-afternoon. However, keep in mind that exercise – at any time of the day – is best. So if you have tried early-morning exercise and it did not work for you, don't worry. You will accomplish your goals regardless of the time of day you exercise.

Use a variety of machines. If you are using indoor cardiovascular machines, stay on the same machine for a maximum of 10 to 15 minutes. This will create better muscle balance. I would rather see someone spend 10 minutes each on the StairMaster™, rowing machine, treadmill and ski machine than spend 40 minutes just on the StairMaster. If you are using the same machine or doing the same activity all the time, the muscles targeted with this exercise will continue to get fitter but other, neglected muscles will not, and muscle imbalances are sure to appear. A varied method of training will develop a more toned physique overall and reduce your risk for injury.

In addition, you might find that you can maintain a higher intensity by mixing up your workout. Although you are using many of the same muscles during many of the indoor activities, they are being used in a slightly different way. You might find that if you stay on the same machine you might start to get tired and have to reduce the intensity of your workout, whereas by quickly jumping onto another machine, you might be able to work hard again. And, finally, mixing up your indoor machines will also help to prevent boredom. I have no difficulty going for a two-hour bike ride outside, but get me on a stationary bike and after 10 minutes I am stir-crazy!

Schedule at least one recovery day into your weekly exercise program. Remember this: Muscle tissue does not grow stronger during exercise. In fact, muscle breaks down during exercise! It needs a period of recovery to repair, grow, develop and get stronger. Back-to-back hard workouts never give the muscles a chance to fully recover. Incorporating one to two recovery days into your weekly workout schedule will ensure your body gets a chance to heal. Do not think, however, that you need to stay home, chained to your couch and TV. When I say "recovery," I mean that maybe you go for an easy stroll or hike or cycle but you are not concerned about getting into your training zone. These are the days you get to just enjoy life and take time to experience its simpler pleasures.

HOMEWORK

It is time to design your fine-tuned cardiovascular program. Review your Personal Exercise Program and consider all the tips we have just discussed. Incorporate an easy, moderate and hard workout each week, include a warm-up and cool-down with each workout, and try a cardio-split workout once or twice each week. Remember also to consider your lifestyle. How many days per week do you think you could commit to? What time of the day works best for you? Which days will work best to exercise and which to take as rest days? After looking at all these variables, take your three primary aerobic activities and program them into an ideal workout week using the schedule below.

SAMPLE PERSONAL EXERCISE PROGRAM

MON.	TUES.	WED.	THURS.	FRI.	SAT.	SUN.
Run 30 minutes at an RPE intensity of 6 to 7	Indoor workout 60 minutes (10 minutes on six different machines) at an RPE intensity of 5	Rest	Outdoor bike ride 40 minutes at an RPE intensity of 6 to 7	Run 20 minutes at an RPE intensity of 8	Cardio-split: Morning power walk 75 minutes at an RPE intensity of 5 Evening in-line skate 45 minutes at an RPE intensity of 5	Rest

IDEAL PERSONAL EXERCISE PROGRAM

MON.	TUES.	WED.	THURS.	FRI.	SAT.	SUN.

When designing programs, it is imperative that you set an ideal and a maintenance goal. For example, your ideal cardiovascular goal might be five workouts per week, but your maintenance goal will take into consideration weeks when you are really busy at work or away on holidays. This will prevent you from getting off track and backsliding. Your maintenance or minimal goal is the minimum exercise you will commit to even if life is going rough. This will ensure you maintain your present level of fitness. Generally, if you get in one good, high-intensity cardio activity in a week when life is tough, you will maintain your fitness. Take the time now to record your ideal cardiovascular goal and your maintenance cardiovascular goal.

IDEAL GOAL   MAINTENANCE GOAL

_____   _____

THE 20-MINUTE MYTH

DO I NEED TO EXERCISE FOR AT LEAST 20 MINUTES BEFORE FAT LOSS KICKS IN?

After about 20 minutes of exercise, the brain signals a sudden release of fats into the bloodstream. This has led many people to mistakenly believe that you only start burning fat after 20 minutes of exercise. This is not true. In fact, as I said earlier, you are always burning fat, even right now while reading this book. As soon as you start to exercise, your muscles request energy. Since the fat cells are already releasing fat, they do not get too excited about the request. But after about 20 minutes, the fat cells realize you mean business and your muscles definitely need more energy, so they release more fat. But remember, you are always burning fat. Even though you might be less efficient at using fat in the first 20 minutes of exercise, you are still burning calories and, therefore, mobilizing and utilizing fat. Caloric expenditure is the key variable for fat loss.

Even if you did only burn sugar during an activity, once the activity was finished, your body would start to burn fat to assist with its recovery. Fat provides the energy required to assist in the replenishment of the treasured sugar stores and other fuels and to help the body recover from the intense activity. Fat is always the predominant fuel used during the recovery phase, so if you have just experienced an intense exercise bout, more recovery will be required and more fat will be utilized.

> PEOPLE WHO DO NOT EXPERIENCE SELF-LOVE HAVE LITTLE OR NO CAPACITY TO LOVE OTHERS.
>
> NATHANIEL BRANDEN

MEASURING INTENSITY

Many exercisers question whether they are working too hard or should be breaking more of a sweat. How do you know if you are exercising in the right intensity zones? That is where monitoring your heart rate comes in. Traditionally an intensity of 70 percent of your maximum heart rate was thought to be the ideal. But this one-size-fits-all approach might not provide the best results for everyone. We are finding that a more custom-designed approach is more effective. Here is how to go about it.

First, you have to determine which of the following zones fits your goals: general health, weight management, aerobic conditioning, advanced conditioning or a combination of all four.

Zone 1: General health. A great deal of research indicates that being active at 50 to 60 percent of your maximum heart rate, consistently and for a total of 30 minutes on most days, reduces the risk of developing many chronic diseases. Low-intensity activities such as walking, gardening, performing household chores or cycling at an easy pace will achieve this. If someone does not need to lose body fat and is not training for a sporting event, this may be all they need to do to stay healthy.

MAN ALONE
IS THE ARCHITECT
OF HIS DESTINY.
THE GREATEST
REVOLUTION
IN MY GENERATION
IS THAT HUMAN
BEINGS, BY
CHANGING THE
INNER ATTITUDES
OF THE MIND,
CAN CHANGE
THE OUTER
ASPECTS
OF THEIR
LIVES.

WILLIAM
JAMES

Zone 2: Weight management. If your goal is to reduce body fat and you have been relatively inactive, you will need to train at a level of 60 to 70 percent of your maximum heart rate. This is still within your comfort zone and allows you to exercise at a steady pace for a long enough time to burn off a substantial number of calories.

Zone 3: Aerobic conditioning/weight management. If your goal is to improve your cardiovascular conditioning for better stamina and endurance, you should train within a zone of 70 to 80 percent of your maximum heart rate. This is also a good zone for fat burning if you are already fairly fit. This zone represents a more vigorous level of activity than zones 1 or 2.

Zone 4: Advanced conditioning. If you are in top shape and training for a sporting event such as a race, a triathlon or tennis, you might need to include some workouts at 80 percent or more of your maximum heart rate. This level of training is both physically and mentally demanding, so it is not something you would do on a daily basis. And it is not for everyone. Only the really fit should consider working in this range. This zone is also a fat-burning zone if you are extremely fit.

Ideally, your exercise program will include workouts in each of these zones – long and easy to short and hard. So how do you determine whether you're in the right zone during any given workout? Here is a formula to help you figure it all out.

- *Estimated maximum heart rate (MHR):*
  Females = 226 – your age
  Males = 220 – your age

- *Low end of training zone = MHR x lower percentage*

- *High end of training zone = MHR x higher percentage*

This age-adjusted maximum heart rate formula is perfect for our purposes. A more accurate method is to determine your maximum heart rate in a laboratory setting using a stress test facilitated by a physician or sports physiologist. The tests are generally administered on a treadmill or exercise bicycle and cost anywhere between $100 and $300. Assuming you don't want to spend the money on a maximal heart rate test, here's how to figure out your heart rate zones without the fancy equipment.

Let us take as an example a 40-year-old inactive woman who wants to lose body fat. The majority of her workouts will be in zone 2 (60 to 70 percent of MHR).

- *Estimated maximum heart rate (MHR) = 226 – age (40) = 186*

- *Low end of training zone = MHR (186) x 60% = 112 beats per minute*

- *High end of training zone = MHR (186) x 70% = 130 beats per minutes*

Doing the math, we see she needs to train at a heart rate of 112 to 130 beats per minute (bpm).

WE CAN
DO ANYTHING
WE WANT TO
DO IF WE
STICK WITH
IT LONG
ENOUGH.

HELEN
KELLER

HOMEWORK

1. Determine your estimated maximum heart rate.

- *Females: MHR = 226 – your age   = _____*

  or
- *Males: MHR = 220 – your age   = _____*

2. Determine which of the four training zones you'd like to calculate

- *Zone _____ = _____ % to _____ %*

3. Determine the low end of your training zone.

- *Low end of training zone =*
  MHR (_____) x _____% = _____ bpm

4. Determine the high end of your training zone.

- *High end of training zone =*
  MHR (_____) x _____% = _____ bpm

5. According to this formula, your optimal training zone is a range of _____ to _____ beats per minute.

A MORE ACCURATE HEART RATE FORMULA

If you take the time to determine your true resting heart rate, your heart rate zones will be more on target. To determine your true resting heart rate, before you get up in the morning, measure your heart rate for one minute. Be sure to wait a few minutes after your alarm has gone off, so your heart will have recovered from being startled. Do this three days in a row and take the average of all three numbers. This is your resting heart rate (RHR).

HOMEWORK

1. Determine and record your true resting heart rate.

- *Day 1: _____ beats per minute*

- *Day 2: _____ beats per minute*

- *Day 3: _____ beats per minute*

- *Total: _____ ÷ 3 = average resting heart rate (RHR) of _____ bpm*

Now complete the following formula. Let's do a sample run-through first. Let's take the example of a 40-year-old inactive woman who wants to lose body fat. Let's say we've determined that her resting heart rate in the morning is 70 beats per minute (bpm).

APPLY
DISCIPLINE
TO YOUR
THOUGHTS WHEN
THEY BECOME
ANXIOUS OVER
THE OUTCOME
OF A GOAL.
IMPATIENCE
BREEDS
ANXIETY, FEAR,
DISCOURAGEMENT
AND FAILURE.
PATIENCE CREATES
CONFIDENCE,
DECISIVENESS
AND RATIONAL
OUTLOOK, WHICH
EVENTUALLY
LEADS TO
SUCCESS.

BRIAN
ADAMS

- *Her estimated maximum heart rate (MHR)*
  = 226 – age (40) = 186

- *Low end of training zone = [MHR (186) – RHR (70 bpm)*
  x 60%] + 70 bpm = 140 bpm

- *High end of training zone = (MHR (186) – RHR (70 bpm)*
  x 70%] + 70 bpm = 151 bpm

Doing the math, we see she actually needs to train at a heart rate of 140 to 151 beats per minute rather than the previously calculated 112 to 130 beats per minute.

2. Determine your estimated maximum heart rate using this more accurate formula.

- *Females: MHR = 226 – your age   = _____*
  or
- *Males: MHR = 220 – your age   = _____*

3. Determine which of the four training zones you'd like to calculate:

- *Zone _____ = _____ % to   _____ %*

4. Determine the low end of your training zone.

- *Low end of training zone = [MHR (_____) – RHR (_____)*
  x _____%] + RHR (_____) = _____ beats per minute

5. Determine the high end of your training zone:

- *High end of training zone = [MHR (_____) – RHR (_____)*
  x _____%] + RHR = _____ beats per minute

6. Your more accurate optimal training zone is a range of _____ to _____ beats per minute.

Once you have determined your optimal training zones for each workout, the best way to ensure that you are in the correct zone is to invest in a heart rate monitor. This will allow you to accurately and quickly analyze your heart rate and easily intensify or reduce the intensity of your workout if you are not in the right zone. Unfortunately, manual heart rate monitoring (on your wrist or neck) has been found to be inaccurate, with errors as high as 27 beats per minute. In addition, when testing on your neck or wrist, you have to stop and interrupt your workout to do the reading.

Although I regularly use battery-operated heart rate monitors with my clients, they do have their drawbacks. One, you might not want to invest the cash, and two, your heart rate

can be affected by variables such as food, medication, temperature and stress. So it is necessary to monitor the intensity
of your workouts with an additional indicator, the rating of
perceived exertion (RPE) scale.

A NEW SCALE TO MEASURE INTENSITY

Rating of Perceived Exertion (RPE) is a scale that calls on
your own perception of the intensity of a workout to indicate
whether you are training in the appropriate zone. RPE is
gaining popularity because of its effectiveness, simplicity and
safety. The RPE scale was developed by Dr. Gunnar Borg
of Sweden. Borg noticed a close relationship between an
athlete's exercising heart rate (which is directly related to the
intensity of the exercise) and how the athlete actually
perceived his or her effort. The original Borg method used a
scale from 6 to 20. This has since been modified, to a more
user-friendly scale of 0 to 10. Zero on the scale represents a
resting level, with no elevation in breathing. At the other
extreme, a rating of 10 indicates all-out effort and severe
exhaustion. Here is how the RPE scale breaks down so you
know how to rate your workouts.

0 – Represents a resting level, with no elevation in your breathing.

1 – Represents a more active rest, like working at your desk, with
no elevation in your breathing.

2 – Represents an active resting level, like getting dressed or walking around in your house, with no elevation in your breathing.

3 – Represents a low level of activity, like gardening or the warm-
up stages in a workout. You may be aware of your breathing,
but it is slow and natural.

4 – Represents a low level of activity, like a stroll or an easy bike ride, with a slight elevation in
breathing. You are still well within your comfort zone. This would be your predominant
training zone if you were exercising in the general health training zone.

5 – Represents a moderate level of activity like walking briskly. Your breathing is more elevated
than in level 4, but you are still well within your comfort zone. This would be your predominant training zone if you were exercising in the weight management training zone or if you
were scheduled for a long, easy workout.

6 – Represents a moderate level of activity, like walking briskly to a very late appointment. Your
breathing is faster and deeper but you are still at a level that is within your comfort zone.
You feel that you can comfortably hold a conversation. This would still be your weight
management training zone or your moderate-intensity workout zone.

A PESSIMIST
IS VERY
GLOOMY AND
DEPRESSED,
LAZY AND
LETHARGIC.
CHEERFULNESS IS
UNKNOWN TO
HIM. HE INFECTS
OTHERS.
PESSIMISM IS
AN EPIDEMIC
AND INFECTIOUS
DISEASE. A
PESSIMIST CANNOT
SUCCEED IN
THE WORLD.

SIVANANDA

THERE IS
NO USE
WHATSOEVER
TRYING TO
HELP PEOPLE
WHO DO NOT
HELP THEMSELVES.
YOU CANNOT
PUSH ANYONE
UP A LADDER
UNLESS HE IS
WILLING TO
CLIMB
HIMSELF.

ANDREW
CARNEGIE

7 – Represents a vigorous level of activity, like jogging. Your breathing is more rapid and deep, and you feel as if you could hold a conversation but would probably prefer not to. This intensity is beginning to feel more challenging and outside of your comfort zone. This would be your predominant training zone if you were exercising in the aerobic conditioning/weight management zone or were performing a moderate-intensity workout.

8 – Represents a vigorous level of activity, like faster running. You can hold a conversation but it would be short. You think you can continue for the remainder of your session, but you are not 100 percent confident that you can make it. You feel that you are outside of your comfort zone and being heavily challenged. This would still be your aerobic conditioning/weight management training zone.

9 – Represents a very, very vigorous level of activity, like sprinting intervals in a run. Your breathing is very laboured, and you could not hold a conversation. You would definitely feel fatigued and outside of your comfort zone. This would be your predominant training zone if you were exercising in the advanced conditioning zone or were performing a short, hard workout.

10 – Represents an all-out effort with severe exhaustion. It is not recommended that you train at this level.

HOMEWORK

Review your Ideal Personal Exercise Program and rate each workout on the RPE scale. Are you exercising in the right zones for your stated goals?

SAME OLD, SAME OLD

At some point in your fat loss exercise program, you are going to find that you are no longer experiencing significant results. This is a very common scenario that most athletes and exercise enthusiasts are faced with.

If you want to change something, you've got to change something. Makes sense, doesn't it? If you follow the same program for a long period of time, your body will adapt. You are eventually going to have to do something different, something your body is not used to, something to "shock" your body into burning more calories. This is the principle of overload that all personal trainers follow when designing personalized exercise programs. It simply states that in order for your body to experience results, it needs to be challenged slightly more than it is used to. If not, your body will plateau and will no longer continue to progress. If you want to continually see results, you will have to continually overload the body just as it begins to plateau. This means changing your program every four to eight weeks.

Avoiding physical plateaus is one benefit of cross-training – not to mention that all the new activities help to minimize boredom, enhance motivation and increase exercise adherence. So the program you have just designed for yourself is only going to be effective for the next few months, and then you are going to have to change things around, try a new activity and just shake things up. Put a reminder in your calendar that will trigger you to make some adjustments to your program.

Do not feel bad if you felt that this section was a lot to absorb. It was! But it is one of the most important components of your fat loss exercise program, so we needed to spend some time clarifying issues and clearing up any misconceptions.

It's important to realize that you do not need to incorporate all of my suggestions into your program today. You might start by just committing to exercising three times per week. Once you have made that a habit, you could perhaps start mixing up the intensity zones by incorporating one easy, one moderate and one hard workout each week. A few months later you could try a cardio-split program. A few months after that, you could invest in a heart rate monitor and start seriously monitoring your heart rate zones. The beauty of this program is that you have designed it. You are your own personal trainer, and at any time you can modify, restructure or adjust your program depending on your success, enjoyment and adherence. For now, feel free to take a break and come back when you are ready to absorb some more material.

PEOPLE WHO POSTPONE HAPPINESS ARE LIKE CHILDREN WHO TRY CHASING RAINBOWS IN AN EFFORT TO FIND THE POT OF GOLD AT THE RAINBOW'S END. . . . YOUR LIFE WILL NEVER BE FULFILLED UNTIL YOU ARE HAPPY HERE AND NOW.

KEN KEYES JR.

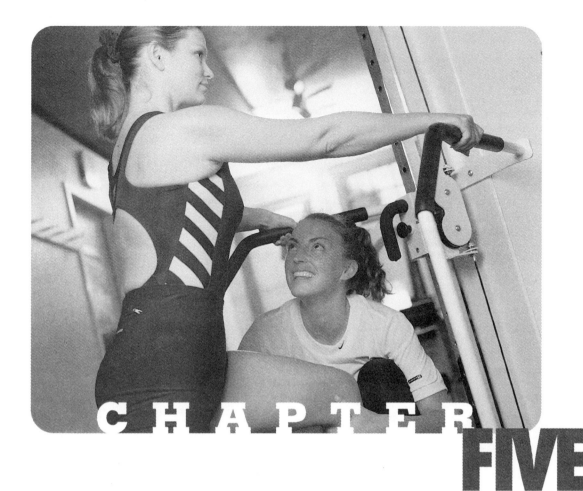

CHAPTER FIVE

Most of us know that exercise is important, but we tend to equate it with aerobic activity like jogging, walking, swimming or cycling. We often forget that resistance training offers just as many health benefits as aerobic exercise. You can expect to experience the following benefits after initiating a resistance training program.

- *improved posture*
- *increased bone density*
- *reduced risk for injury*
- *increased muscular strength and endurance*
- *improved muscle tone*
- *increased fat loss*
- *increased metabolic rate*

MORE MUSCLE EQUALS LESS FAT

Imagine the following effects on an individual's metabolism. During the day your body expends energy to sustain life (basal metabolic rate); to respond to food intake, changes in temperature, or to stress, fear, drugs or hormones; and to undertake physical activity. This daily energy output breaks down by category into 70 percent, 20 percent and 10 percent, respectively. If you can even slightly affect the basal metabolic rate, you might significantly affect the daily calories expended. Remember that the average-sized person burns 1 kcal/min. at rest. If the resting metabolic rate can be increased by just 10 percent, this equates to a rate of 1.1 kcal/min. Doesn't sound like a big deal, does it? But over an hour, this equals an extra six calories, and over a day, an extra 144 calories. Remember that to burn a pound of fat you need to expend 3,500 calories more than you eat. At the basal metabolic rate of 1.1 kcal/min., it would take 24 days (3,500 ÷ 144) to burn one pound (0.45 kg) of extra fat – and this does not include any calories expended through exercise. This amounts to about 15 pounds (6.8 kg) of fat that could be lost in one year by merely raising the basal metabolic rate by 10 percent. I hope this has convinced you to put some muscle on your body.

As we get older, our metabolism – the amount of calories we burn at rest – drops. This is related to a decline in the activity of our liver, kidneys and other organs. This declining rate of activity is almost entirely out of our control – almost. Examine the following chart, which breaks down our metabolism.

BASAL METABOLIC RATE

ORGAN	METABOLIC RATE (KCAL/KG/DAY)	ORGAN WEIGHT (KG)	METABOLIC RATE (KCAL/DAY)	% OF BASAL ENERGY EXPENDITURE
Brain	260	1.4	365	21
Heart	600	0.3	180	20
Kidney	400	0.3	120	7
Liver	359	1.6	560	32
Lungs	200	0.8	160	9
Muscle		40% of total body weight		24

You can see that although your liver activity makes up the highest percentage of metabolic activity, there is really nothing you can do about that. We know that it is in our best interest to keep our metabolism revving, but we can't say, "All right, I need to increase my metabolic rate, so I am going to get my liver in shape. Let's go, liver, start working for me!" In contrast, we can do something about our muscle activity, which contributes 24 percent to our metabolic rate. Muscle comprises approximately 40 percent of our total body weight. If you can get your muscles working at a higher level, the difference to your metabolic rate will be significant.

By developing your muscular system, you will increase your metabolism. Muscle is an energy-burning tissue and thus, the more of it you have on your body, the more fat you will burn both during exercise and during rest. How would you like to be sitting in front of the TV knowing you are burning more fat than you were before you started resistance training? In fact, one pound (0.45 kg) of muscle tissue expends an additional 30 to 40 kilocalories per day. That does not sound like a lot, but consider that after an eight- to 12-week resistance training program, you can expect to develop three to four pounds of lean muscle tissue. That equates to an extra 90 to 160 calories being burned per day. Multiply this by 365 days per year and we are talking about 10 to 14 pounds of fat per year either lost or not gained compared to not having that muscle mass. Now, that is motivation to get into the weight room.

We also know that, on average, we will lose three to five percent of our muscle mass per decade after the age of 25. In fact, the average sedentary 80-year-old man will have lost approximately 50 percent of his |muscle mass. As a result, our fat mass will increase. If you want to reduce the magnitude of this age-related fat gain, start resistance training and depositing muscle on your body.

The difference of having more muscle on our body is even more significant during exercise. The difference in energy expended by a resting compared to a working muscle is quite noticeable. When you start exercising, your muscles demand that your organs and tissues kick into action at a very high rate. If you have more muscle demanding more energy, your caloric expenditure will skyrocket! One study compared the energy costs of treadmill walking between obese and lean, highly muscular men who were the same weight and height. The results showed that the energy expenditure was significantly higher at any given speed and grade of walking for the body builders compared to the obese males. Expenditure reached up to 100 calories higher for the muscular men at a moderate walking pace up an incline. These results demonstrate that just by having more muscle on your body, you will burn more energy both during exercise and at rest.

> THOUGHTS OF STRENGTH BOTH BUILD STRENGTH FROM WITHIN AND ATTRACT IT FROM WITHOUT. THOUGHTS OF WEAKNESS ACTUALIZE WEAKNESS FROM WITHIN AND ATTRACT IT FROM WITHOUT.
>
> RALPH W. TRINE

The American College of Sports Medicine recommends one set of eight to 12 (10 to 15 if you are 50 years or older) repetitions for each major muscle group two times a week to improve overall muscle conditioning. This recommendation is also sufficient to maximize fat loss.

Here are some definitions that may help to clarify this component of your program.

- *A repetition (or rep) refers to the number of times you perform an exercise without stopping.*

- *A set refers to the number of times you perform a complete series of repetitions. For example, you might perform two sets of 10 reps.*

Many exercisers, wanting to lose body fat and understanding that gaining muscle is crucial to maximizing fat loss, have made muscle conditioning a priority. However, by spending extra time in the weight room they have sacrificed very important cardiovascular exercise time. It is important to remember that you burn calories and fat directly during aerobic exercise, and this component of your program should be your priority. Muscle conditioning is also a must, but two times per week for 30 to 45 minutes will be sufficient in the beginning to develop your muscles and help rev up your metabolism.

A resistance-training program that does not focus on technique will get you results much more slowly and may put you at risk for injury. Here are some important tips on technique.

- *Quality and execution of movement is critical. It makes no sense to perform 20 sloppy reps. It is far better to perform eight reps with perfect form and then take a break.*

- *Take it slow. Proper resistance training is not a fast sport. Wayne Westcott, a leading strength-and-conditioning researcher, has determined that one repetition should take approximately five to six seconds; that is, two seconds to lift the weight and four seconds to slowly lower the weight in a controlled fashion. Most people lift weights much too quickly, using momentum instead of muscle. A proper set of eight to 12 repetitions should take approximately one minute to complete. Proper execution of each rep is the most important factor in weight training. Reps performed with poor technique will get you nowhere.*

- *Breathe. A proper breathing rhythm will make each set more effective. Focus on exhaling as you lift the weight or when you exert, and inhale as you recover or lower the weight.*

- *Sit up straight. Proper posture is vital to ensure you are working the correct muscle groups and not putting your body at risk for injury. Always keep your abdominals contracted throughout the entire set of any exercise. Pull them up and in toward your spine to help stabilize your trunk. Keep your shoulders back and chest lifted up and out during any seated, bent over or standing exercise.*

> A LOT OF SUCCESSFUL PEOPLE ARE RISK-TAKERS. UNLESS YOU ARE WILLING TO DO THAT, TO HAVE A GO, TO FAIL MISERABLY AND HAVE ANOTHER GO, SUCCESS WON'T HAPPEN.
>
> PHILIP ADAMS

- *A good exercise set will finish just as you hit momentary muscle fatigue. This is the point at which you absolutely cannot do another rep with perfect form. If you can perform more reps, you should either perform the extra reps to hit momentary muscle fatigue or, next time, increase the resistance so you can hit momentary muscle fatigue within the suggested eight to 12 reps.*

- *Never go to failure. Failure is when you continue the set with poor technique or when other muscle groups have kicked in to help you finish the set. It is important that you always avoid bad technique and muscle substitution.*

- *If you cannot perform eight reps, the weight is too heavy. If you can perform 12 reps with perfect technique, increase the weight by five percent.*

- *Perform your muscle-conditioning sessions on alternating days. Do not do these workouts back-to-back. Your muscles require a rest day between these sessions.*

- *Put your mind into it. It is okay to disassociate while performing some fitness activities. For example, you can jump onto a treadmill and punch in a seven-minute-mile pace and, whether you think about it or not, you will expend the same amount of calories. However, this is not the case with muscle-conditioning exercise. You must focus on what you're doing, because there is such a strong connection between the brain, the nerves and the muscles. We know that if you actually concentrate on what you are doing, you can significantly increase the amount of muscle activity measured during these exercises. So put down your magazine, cease all conversation and really focus on each set. Each repetition and each set will become much more effective, and you will experience results much more quickly.*

> BELIEVE IN YOURSELF; FEEL THAT YOU ARE ABLE TO DOMINATE YOUR SURROUNDINGS. RESOLVE THAT YOU WILL BE MASTER AND NOT THE SLAVE OF CIRCUMSTANCES.
>
> ORISON S. MARDEN

WHICH EXERCISES WILL DO THE TRICK?

There are literally hundreds of different exercises you could perform to get the results you are looking for. Here are a few guidelines to follow when designing your resistance-training program.

Start with basic exercises. It is necessary to progress from exercises that require the least amount of coordination, balance and overall fitness to exercises that maximally challenge these skills. This means that in the beginning, very basic exercises will suffice. As you master the technique of these exercises, you should advance your program by incorporating more challenging exercises.

For example, when performing a chest press, you might start on a machine that has a back support, so all you have to think about is pushing the bar. As you master this skill and your muscle conditioning improves, you can try performing the exercise with hand weights

PERSONAL
SUCCESS IS
NEVER STATIC.
IT USUALLY
COMES IN
SMALL STEPS
LEADING TO
OTHER SMALL
STEPS THAT
LEAD TO
BROADER
ACHIEVEMENT.

WES
ROBERTS

instead. Now you have to think about balancing the hand weights, which adds a new dimension to the movement. Once you have mastered this skill, you can progress to performing the exercise lying over an exercise ball instead of on a bench. Now, not only do you have to think about the hand weights, you also have to consider that you are now lying on a moveable object, which will add a further challenge to the exercise.

You can follow this type of progression for any exercise. Every four to eight weeks, try to add a new challenge to any exercise you are performing. But it is always important that you follow the appropriate gradual progression. You definitely do not want to attempt more challenging exercises without having first developed the basic foundation for the skill.

Change your program regularly. The only perfect resistance-training program is one that changes. A program that we design today might be perfect today, but in four to eight weeks, it will no longer be perfect or effective. We know that the body needs to be challenged in order to progress. A plateau will occur once the body adapts to any program. If you want continued results, you need to change your program every four to eight weeks, in order to constantly challenge your body and force it to respond in a positive fashion. You can change your program in various ways. You can change the amount of weight you lift, the exercises you perform, the order in which you perform the exercises, the number of sets or reps you do, the amount of recovery time you take between exercises, the number of days you work out each week . . .

This is where investing in the services of a personal trainer might save you a lot of time. It is not necessary for you to spend a fortune on a consultation. Even one or two sessions every two months, in order to make the changes required for you to see continued results, will help you get the most from your workout time. You also don't need to purchase a gym membership; many personal trainers will come to you and design a home program that you can follow. IDEA, the International Health and Fitness Source, released a statistic recently at one of its international conferences. It stated that only 25 percent of people working out are getting the results they want. But out of the 25 percent of people getting results, 90 percent of them are working with a personal trainer. So it is quite clear that having a personal coach to monitor your progress and update your program regularly is an investment in your health worth making.

Here are some exercises that you can start today and perform in the privacy of your own home. You will need to purchase one to two exercise tubes with handles and a set of hand weights (or you can use soup cans), available at any fitness or sporting goods retailer. You will also need access to a fixed pole (such as a gate, fence, house or bedpost), a sturdy chair, a staircase and a ball.

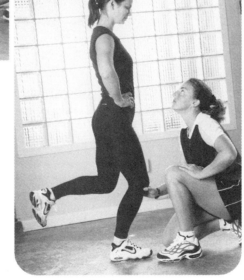

starting position

Practise each of the exercises below, following the tips on proper technique listed.

1.a.

KNEE DIP,
a beginner
exercise
for thighs
and buttocks
(quadriceps,
hamstrings
and gluteus
muscles)

finishing position

Beginner – A lunge exercise is too advanced for you at this point. Instead, perform a knee dip. Stand on one leg with perfect posture. Keep your weight distributed on all four corners of your foot and keep your knee pointed forward throughout the entire exercise. Slowly, bending at your knee, lower your body weight down just a few inches. Keep your body balanced and controlled throughout the entire exercise. Return to the starting position. Complete eight to 15 reps for each leg.

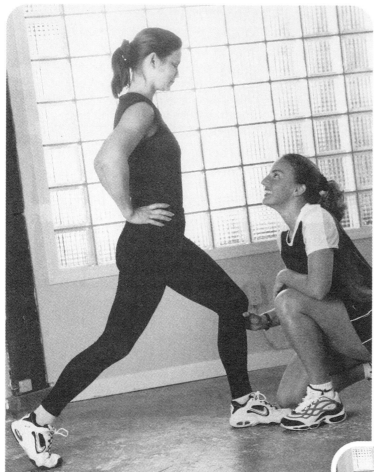

starting position

1.b.

LUNGE,
an intermediate
/advanced
exercise for
thighs and
buttocks
(quadriceps,
hamstrings and
gluteus muscles)

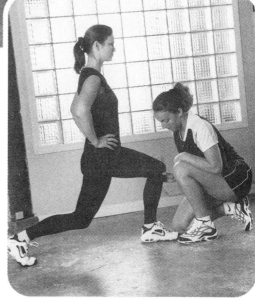

finishing position

Intermediate – Stand with one leg positioned in front of the other leg. Keep the front knee over top of the ankle. Keep the back knee underneath or slightly behind your hips. Slowly lower the back knee toward the ground, keeping the front knee over top of the ankle the entire time. Keep your body weight positioned over the front leg – this is your working leg. Maintain proper posture and keep your abdominals contracted. Complete eight to 15 reps for each leg.

Advanced – Perform the same exercise as above but start to add resistance by holding free weights in your arms, held relaxed at your sides.

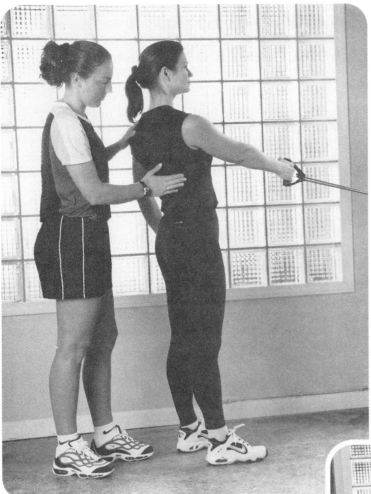

intermediate starting position

2.

MID ROW, for mid-back muscles (rhomboids, middle trapezius and lattisimus dorsi)

Beginner – Wrap your tube around a fixed pole at about shoulder height. Holding one handle in each hand, pull back with your arms (like rowing a boat) to strengthen your back. Keep your shoulders square to the pole and pull your elbows back as far as you comfortably can. Squeeze your shoulder blades into the middle of your back. Perform eight to 15 reps.

Intermediate – Do the exercise as above but hold both handles in one hand so you are performing a single-arm row. Perform eight to 15 reps for each arm.

Advanced – Do the same exercise as above but wrap two tubes around the pole so you are holding four handles in one hand.

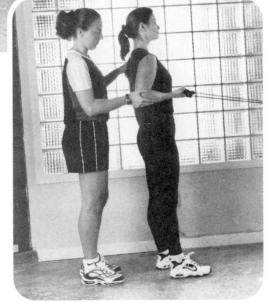

finishing position

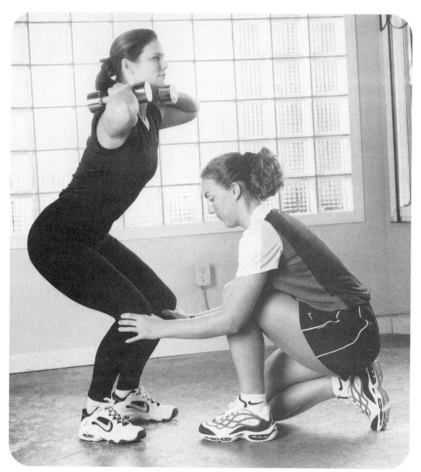

intermediate/advanced position

3.

SQUATS,
for thighs
and buttocks
(quadriceps,
hamstrings
and gluteus
muscles)

Beginner – Start by sitting in a chair. Maintain proper posture by keeping your abdominals contracted and your chest up and shoulders back. Keep your kneecaps facing forward and your feet about shoulder width apart. Now slowly stand up and then slowly lower to the starting position. Perform eight to 15 repetitions.

Intermediate – Perform the same exercise as above but without the chair (i.e., from a squat) and holding light hand weights.

Advanced – Increase the amount of weight you are holding.

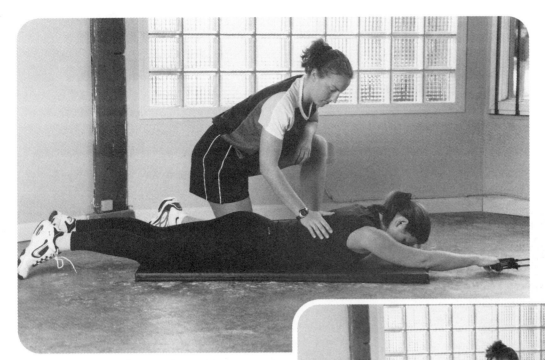

intermediate starting position

finishing position

4.

LAT PULL-DOWNS,
for back
muscles
(lattisimus
dorsi)

Beginner – Wrap an exercise tube around a pole. Lie flat on your stomach and hold one handle in each hand. Now slowly pull the tubes so that your elbows travel beside your body and finish at your waist. Now slowly return to your starting position. Perform eight to 15 reps for each arm.

Intermediate – Perform the same exercise as above but hold both handles in one hand and pull. Position the other hand underneath your head.

Advanced – Perform the same exercise as above but wrap two tubes around the pole and hold all four handles in one hand.

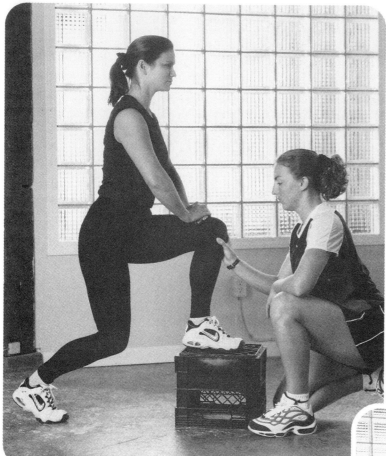

intermediate starting position

5.

STEP-UPS,
for thighs
and buttocks
(quadriceps,
hamstrings
and gluteus
muscles)

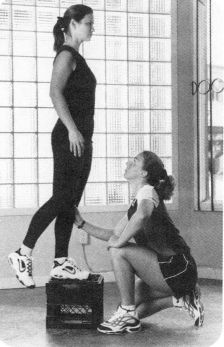

finishing position

Beginner – Position yourself in front of a staircase with one foot on the bottom step. Keep your kneecap facing forward and your weight distributed on all four corners of your foot. Now slowly step up, extending the supporting knee into a fully upright, balanced position. Now slowly lower your leg down to the starting position. Perform eight to 15 reps for each leg.

Intermediate – Perform the same exercise as above but in the downward position, finish in a deeper lunge.

Advanced – Perform the same exercise as above but increase the height of the step or hold hand weights to increase the resistance.

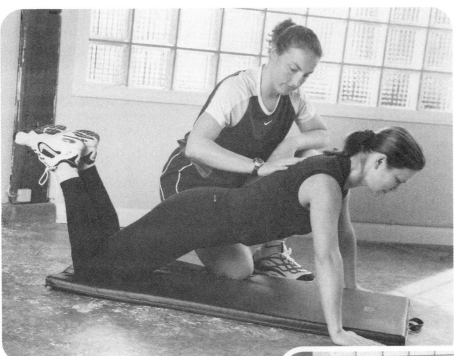

intermediate starting position

6.

PUSH-UPS,
for chest muscles
(pectorals) and
muscles at the
back of the
arm (triceps)

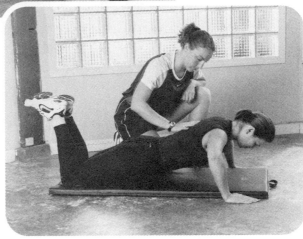

finishing position

Beginner – Lie on your stomach. Position your hands on the floor a few inches away from your shoulders. Make sure that your elbows are directly over top or to the inside of your wrists. Keep your abdominals contracted and your back in a neutral position. Now use your hands to slowly push yourself up from your knees and slowly lower yourself down to the starting position. Relax for a few seconds. Repeat the exercise. Perform eight to 15 reps with a break between each one.

Intermediate – Perform the same exercise as above but without taking a rest between reps.

Advanced – Perform the same exercise as above but from your toes instead of your knees.

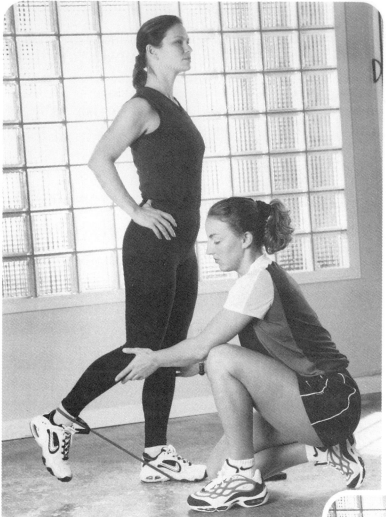

intermediate starting position

7.

HAMSTRING CURLS, for muscles at the back of the thigh (hamstrings)

Beginner – Pull one handle through the other to create a loop in the exercise tube. Wrap the loop around your ankle. Stand on the other end of the tube to anchor it and provide resistance. Holding onto a chair or the wall, keep your legs together and slowly lift the foot with the tube looped around it up toward your buttock. Perform eight to 15 reps for each leg.

Intermediate – Perform the same exercise as above but without holding onto anything.

Advanced – Perform the same exercise as above but with two tubes wrapped around your ankle.

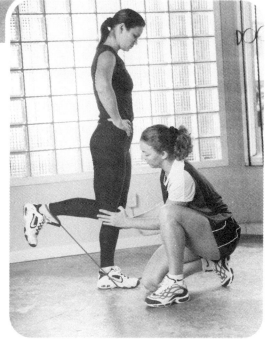

finishing position

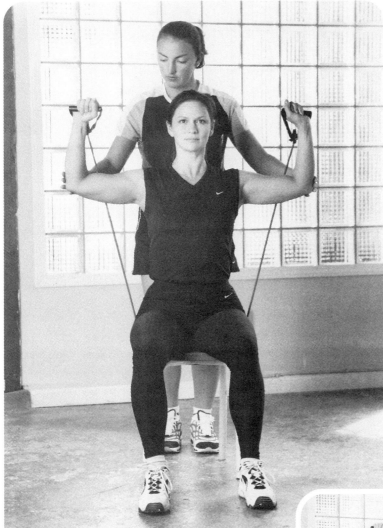

intermediate starting position

8.

OVERHEAD SHOULDER PRESS, for shoulder muscles (deltoids) and muscles at the back of the arm (triceps)

Beginner – Wrap the exercise tube underneath the seat of a chair. Grab both handles and position one arm at about shoulder height at your side and anchor the other arm at your torso. Slowly extend the arm at your shoulder above your head. Maintain proper posture throughout the exercise. Perform eight to 15 reps for each arm.

Intermediate – Perform the same exercise as above but lift both arms overhead at the same time.

Advanced – Perform the same exercise as above but use two tubes.

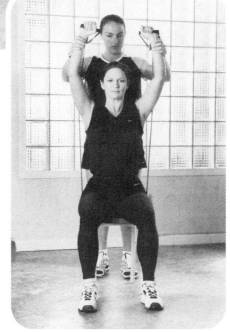

finishing position

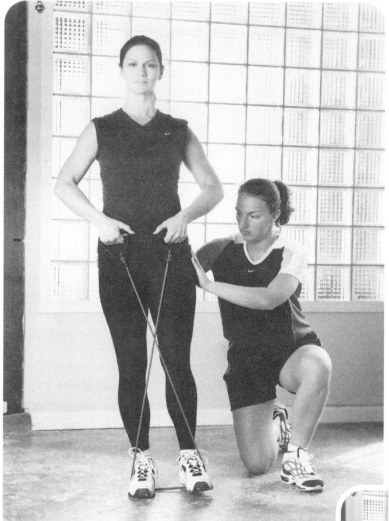

starting position

9.

OUTER THIGH LIFT, for outer thigh muscles (abductors)

Beginner – Hold the exercise handles in each hand and step on the middle of the tube. Keeping your abdominals contracted and maintaining proper posture, slowly lift one leg out to the side. Try not to lean into the supporting leg, and lift the leg only about 30 degrees off the floor. Alternate legs and perform eight to 15 reps for each side.

Intermediate – Perform the same exercise as above but do eight to 15 reps consecutively on one leg, then switch and do the other leg.

Advanced – Perform the same exercise as above but use two tubes.

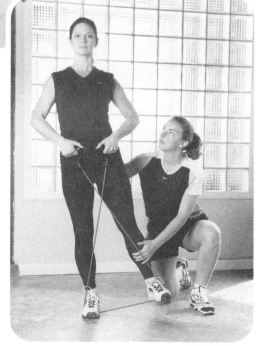

finishing position

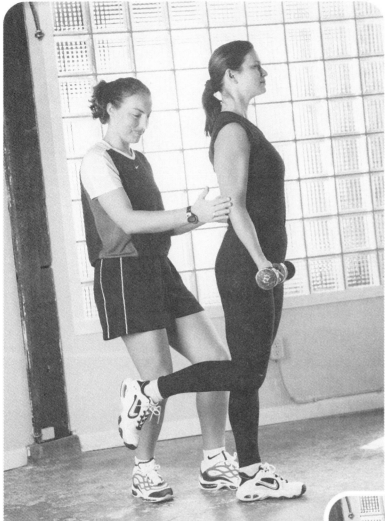

10.

ONE-LEGGED BICEP CURL,
for muscles at the front of the arm (biceps) and balance

intermediate/advanced starting position

Beginner – Position most of your body weight onto one leg but keep the other leg touching the floor to help maintain balance and form. Hold one hand weight in each hand. Maintain perfect posture, chest out and shoulders back, then slowly lift the hand weight up toward your shoulders. Perform eight to 15 reps with your weight on one leg. Take a small break, then perform eight to 15 reps with your weight on the other leg.

Intermediate – Perform the same exercise as above but position yourself completely on one leg.

Advanced – Perform the same exercise as above but increase the amount of weight you are lifting.

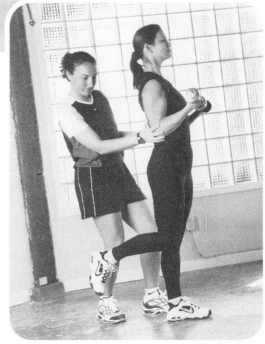

finishing position

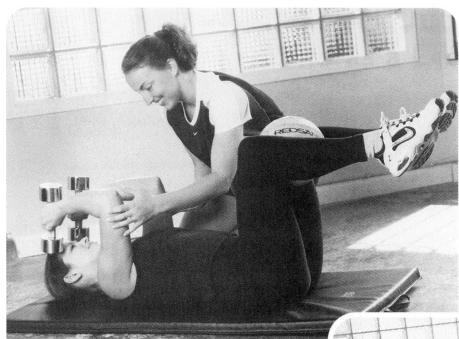
intermediate/advanced starting position

11.

SUPINE INNER THIGH AND TRICEP EXTENSION, for muscles at the back of the arm (triceps) and inner thigh muscles (adductors)

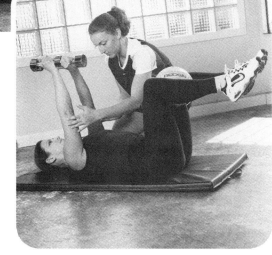
finishing position

Beginner – Lie on your back with your feet positioned on the floor and a ball (soccer ball, volleyball, basketball) positioned between your knees. Maintain a constant contraction in your inner thigh muscles to keep the ball positioned between your legs. Hold a hand weight in each hand and position your arms so they are fully extended over top of your shoulder and all your joints are stacked – the elbow is over the shoulder and the wrist is over the elbow. Keep your elbows positioned over your shoulders as you slowly bend them and your forearms drop toward your forehead. Lower your arms to each side of your head, then return to the starting position. Perform eight to 15 reps.

Intermediate – Perform the same exercise as above but keep your feet off the floor and your legs suspended in the air. Maintain the constant contraction of your inner thigh muscles.

Advanced – Perform the same exercise as above but use heavier hand weights.

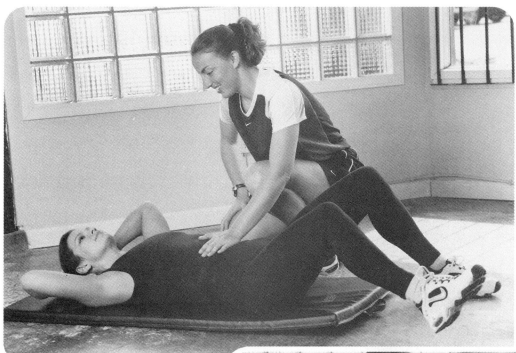

intermediate/advanced starting position

12.

**OBLIQUE
CRUNCHES,**
for side and front
abdominal muscles (external
and internal obliques and
rectus abdominus)

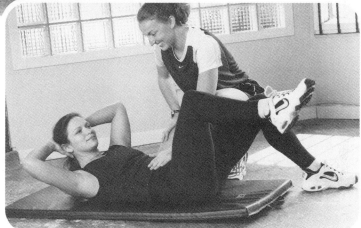

finishing position

Beginner – Lie on your back with your knees bent and your feet positioned on the floor. Place your hands behind your head to lightly support the weight of your head. Keep your chin away from your chest and focus your vision at about 45 degrees from the floor. Avoid looking straight up to the ceiling or toward the opposite wall. Now slowly lift your torso up on an angle. An oblique crunch does not need to involve a large twisting action. Focus on the upward lift on an angle. Contract your abdominals on each repetition. Alternate sides and perform eight to 15 reps on each side.

Intermediate – Perform the same exercise as above but as you lift your upper body, lift the opposite leg at the same time.

Advanced – Perform the same exercise as above but perform all the repetitions on one side and then do the other side.

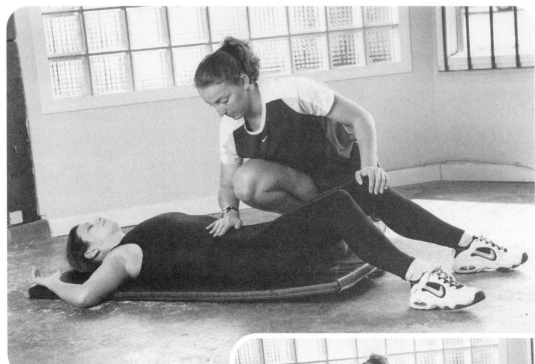

intermediate/advanced starting position

13.

STRAIGHT LEG LIFTS, for abdominal muscles (transverse abdominus and internal and external obliques)

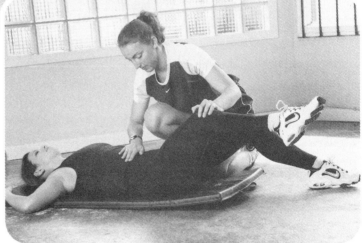

finishing position

Beginner – Lie on your back with your knees bent and your feet positioned on the floor close to your buttocks. Put your hands on your abdominals and pull them in and up so your stomach becomes as flat as you can get it. Keep your stomach in this position throughout the entire exercise as you slowly lift one foot a few inches off the floor. Your back should not move at all during the exercise. Perform eight to 15 reps with each leg.

Intermediate – Perform the same exercise as above but with your legs positioned farther away from your buttocks.

Advanced – Perform the same exercise as above but with your legs straight.

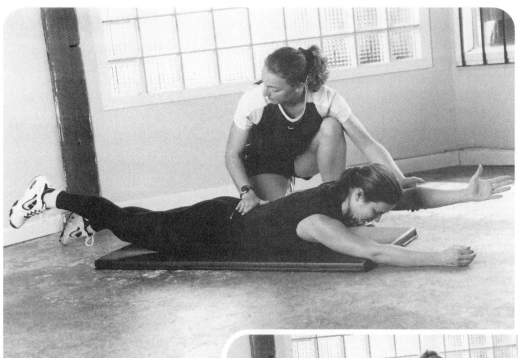

intermediate/advanced starting position

14.

**PRONE ONE-ARM
AND LEG LIFTS,**
for back muscles
(erector spinae)

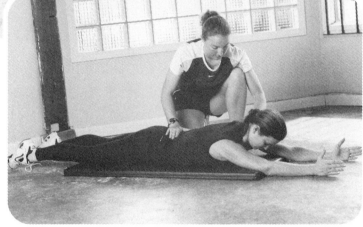

finishing position

Beginner – Lie on your stomach with your abdominals contracted and pulled away from the floor throughout the entire exercise. Start with both arms positioned over your head. Keep your neck in a neutral position. Lift one arm, then lower it. Lift the other arm, then lower it. Lift one leg, then lower it. Lift the other leg, then lower it. Now relax. While lifting your arms and legs, avoid lifting them really high. Instead, focus on reaching with the arms and the legs. Wait a few seconds, then perform the sequence again. Do eight to 15 sequences.

Intermediate – Perform the same exercise as above, but lift the opposite arm and leg simultaneously. Alternate sides and perform eight to 15 reps each side.

Advanced – Perform the same exercise as above, but perform reps for the same side consecutively. Then do the other side.

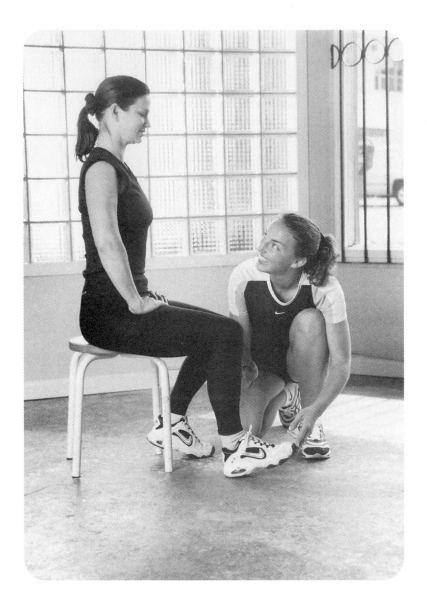

TOE TAPS,
for shin
muscles
(tibialis
anterior)

At least two to three times per week, tap your toes
for about one minute each side to strengthen
your shin muscles.

STRETCH IT OUT

You don't want to develop muscles that are tight and short, so after all workouts, a 10-minute stretch is imperative. Here are some relaxing stretches that you can enjoy after each workout. Hold each stretch for at least 30 seconds – ideally longer. And remember, hold each stretch to the point of tension – not pain.

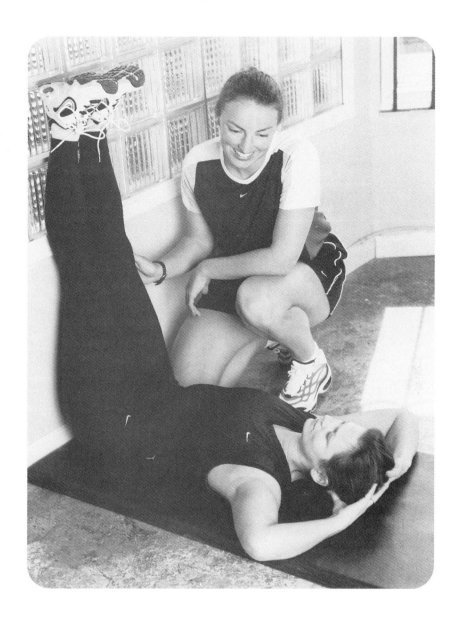

HAMSTRING ON THE WALL

Lie on your back with your hips close to the wall and your legs positioned straight up against the wall. To make the stretch less intense, move your hips a few inches away from the wall. To make the stretch more intense, keep your hips positioned right up against the wall, wrap a towel around your feet and use it to lightly pull your legs a few inches away from the wall. Feel the stretch in the muscles at the back of your upper leg.

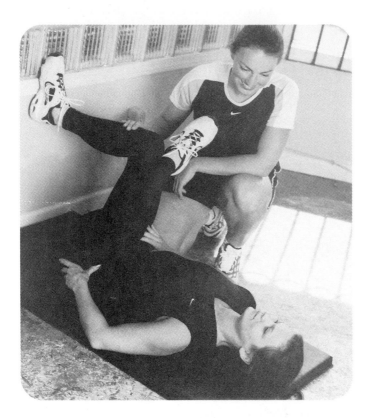

GLUTES ON THE WALL

Lie on your back with your hips positioned farther from the wall. Place one foot on the wall so that the knee bends to 90 degrees. Now place the other ankle onto that thigh. You should feel a light stretch around the outside edge of your hip.

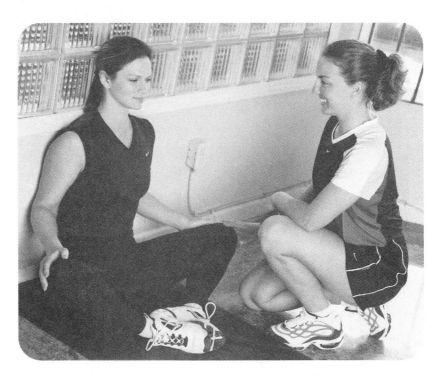

INNER THIGH ON THE WALL

Sit with your back straight up against the wall. Now bring the soles of your feet together and allow your legs to drop out to the side. Feel the stretch through your groin.

HIP FLEXOR STRETCH

Position yourself in a lunge position with your front knee positioned over the front ankle and your back knee positioned comfortably on a mat or towel. Straighten your spine so your posture is fully erect. Lightly press the hip forward. Feel the stretch in the front of your thigh.

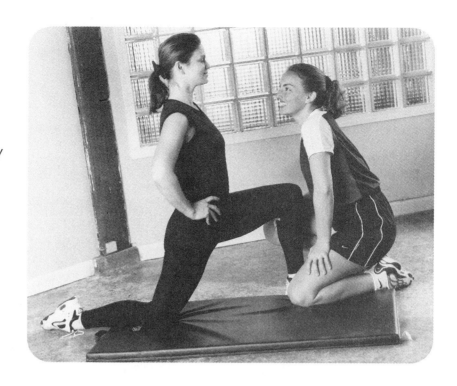

CALF STRETCH

Stand facing a wall. Place one leg close to the wall and the other farther away. Place your hands on the wall. Keep the heel of the back leg positioned firmly into the floor. Feel the stretch in your calf.

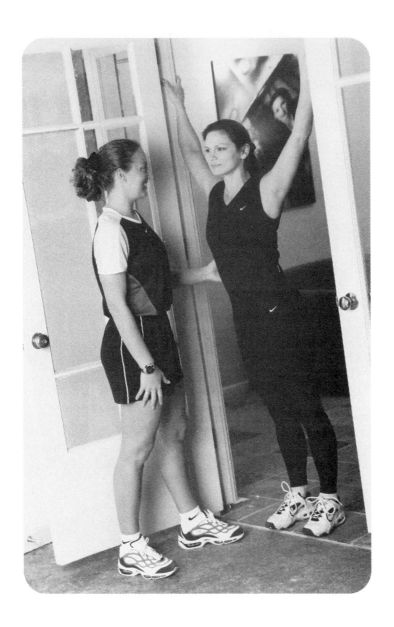

CHEST STRETCH

Stand in a door frame. Place your arms above your head and hold onto the top of the door frame. Now slowly stretch forwards. Next, position your arms at shoulder height in the door frame, then slowly stretch forwards. Next, position your arms below shoulder height in the door frame, then slowly stretch forwards.

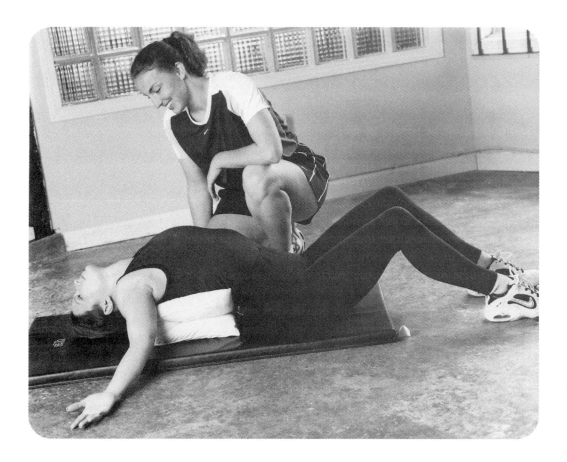

UPPER BACK STRETCH

Place two to three pillows on the floor. Lie on your back with your shoulder blades over the pillows to get a slight arch in your upper back.

HOMEWORK

Decide which two nonconsecutive days during the week you will perform muscle-conditioning exercises. You could do these exercises after one of your aerobic workouts or you could do these exercises (after a warm-up) on a day that you are not doing any aerobic activity. Adjust your Personal Exercise Program accordingly.

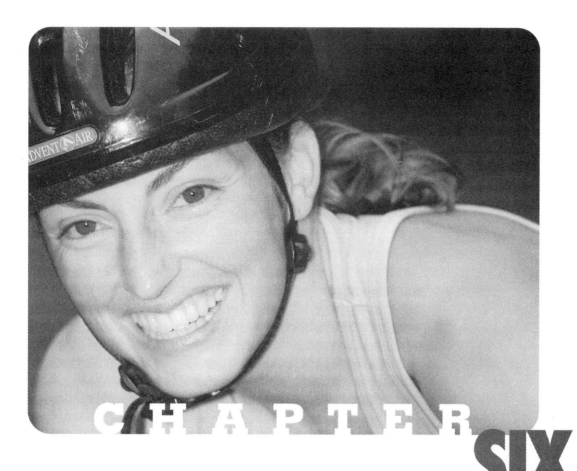

CHAPTER **SIX**

We all know how to eat correctly. In fact, we as a population are much more educated about proper nutrition than we ever have been. But, as we all know too well, knowing how to eat correctly and actually eating correctly are two very different things. There is no trick to eating well to maximize fat loss. It is stuff we have all heard before. Drink lots of water. Eat five small snacks or meals each day. Consume your required intake of fruits, vegetables and whole grain products. Minimize your intake of fat, alcohol and processed foods. There is no special diet or pill that will get you the results you want quickly. But there seems to be a gap between knowing what to do and actually adhering to these simple guidelines.

Obviously, knowledge alone is not power. We all know what we have to do. Only finding the motivation and inspiration to make and adhere to very small changes in our nutrition plan will facilitate success. Finding the motivation to stick to a healthy nutrition plan day in, day out is all it takes. Keeping a Daily Exercise and Nutrition Log and the drills in this chapter will help to motivate and inspire you to make the nutritional changes necessary to maximize fat loss and enhance your health.

With nutrition, I have found that very small changes in someone's eating habits will often bring about big differences. The new habits just need to be consistent and ongoing on a long-term basis.

In this chapter I will provide you with some easy nutrition tips and guide you through designing your own fat loss nutrition program. My philosophy with nutrition is very similar to my take on exercise. If I design your nutrition program for you and tell you that you have to eat broccoli everyday, but you hate broccoli, you are not going to experience any success. You must be involved in the process. It is necessary for you to design a program that you realistically believe you could follow for a lifetime. Remember, I do not believe in any quick fixes. We're talking about a lifelong effort.

WHY DIETS DON'T WORK

How many studies need to prove that diets do not work before our society gets it? The diet industry is still a multibillion-dollar one and continues to thrive despite desperate pleading from leading scientists telling us that diets do not work. We need to wake up and take a dose of reality. If it sounds too good to be true, it probably is!

When you diet, your body actually starts to work against your efforts. As soon as you restrict your caloric intake, your body moves into "famine stage" or "starvation response." Basically, your body does not know when its next meal will be and whether the energy intake will be sufficient for all its internal functions to operate optimally. So, being such an effective piece of machinery, your body slows all internal functions. You move into efficiency mode – a physical slowing down of metabolism. This is absolutely the last thing you want to happen. If you want to maximize fat loss, you want to keep your metabolism revving at a high rate, not at a slow rate. The only way to do this is to eat properly and exercise.

You might notice that after you eat a meal, you feel warmer. The heat comes from digesting your meal. Your liver, pancreas, stomach and intestines have to produce digestive enzymes, which requires energy. Many people who are starting to gain weight conclude that their metabolism might be slowing down and decide to eat less. This depresses their metabolism even more. The point here is that digestion requires energy and will raise your metabolic rate. The key to fat loss is ensuring you are eating regularly enough to raise your metabolic rate to a point where you experience a caloric deficit. Dieting suppresses your metabolic rate. We must avoid this at all costs.

Losing 10 pounds (4.5 kg) is easy. Lock yourself in a closet for a few days and consume just enough water to sustain life. By week's end, you will definitely be 10 pounds lighter. When you are dieting, the scale shows positive confirmation that you are doing the right thing. You definitely start to lose weight. But the problem is, if you are dieting and have lost 10 pounds, you have not lost 10 pounds of fat. Instead, you have lost only two pounds (0.9 kg) of fat, along with three pounds (1.4 kg) of water and five pounds (2.3 kg) of muscle. The muscle loss is the worst thing about quick-weight-loss diets. Muscle is an energy-burning tissue, and when you are dieting, you will lose a whole lot of it. Knowing what you now know about muscles, you can imagine what this does to your ability to burn calories both at rest and during exercise. If fat loss is your goal, you must strive to maintain your muscle mass, as it will keep your metabolism revving at a higher rate.

Studies have also shown that dieting actually makes you less likely to move throughout the day. You sit rather than stand, take an elevator instead of the stairs, fidget less at your desk, so that by the end of the day, even though you have reduced your food intake, you have also reduced your energy output. The bottom line: You lose no body fat.

Dieting also sets restrictions and limitations that are unrealistic and unsustainable in the long run. You will end up bingeing and feeling like a failure.

This brings us to the most serious failure of diets: keeping the weight off. This is clearly the most difficult thing to do. Most people think of diets as a short-term phenomenon, that as soon as they achieve their weight loss goal, they can go back to eating their normal diet. Of course, they inevitably gain all the weight back. When on a diet, a person feels sensations of depression and deprivation. These are emotions they cannot wait to rid of, so their thoughts centre on the day their diet will be over.

A University of California study found that 90 percent of dieters who followed a prescribed diet eventually regained the weight they had lost. Of the 10 percent who were successful in keeping the weight off, 73 percent of them did so just by making better nutrition and lifestyle choices. So when you are deciding on a particular eating plan, ask yourself if you can realistically follow the eating plan for years. If not, stay away from it, because as soon as you stop the plan, you will regain the weight. If a plan imposes strict limits or requires only a few types of foods, be forewarned – it may not be sustainable.

The reality is not new but it bears repeating: The only way to take weight off and keep it off is to exercise regularly and eat nutritiously. It makes sense that if you want to weigh 10 pounds (4.5 kg) less 10 years from now, what counts is what you do over the next 10 years, not over the next six weeks. Short-term restrictive diets set people up for failure. A healthy nutrition plan that you believe you can realistically follow for the rest of your life is the only fat loss nutrition plan that will work.

> EVEN WHEN YOU'RE ON THE RIGHT TRACK, YOU'LL GET RUN OVER IF YOU JUST SIT THERE.
>
> WILL ROGERS

YO-YO DIETING

Many of you might feel very guilty about your previous attempts at dieting. Do not be too hard on yourself. There have been a lot of suggestions that any so-called yo-yo dieting you might have done in the past, during which you lost weight and regained it, will make future attempts at fat loss more difficult. But a review of 43 studies found no convincing evidence to suggest that yo-yo dieting permanently lowers metabolic rate, increases body fat percentage, makes it harder to lose weight next time, raises blood pressure or blood sugar, or increases the risk of dying from heart disease. So whatever has happened in the past does not matter. Your past does not equal your future. In fact, many fitness experts, myself included, believe that you have to go through several attempts or trials before you finally succeed at fat loss.

PURE, DELICIOUS WATER

Did you know that 50 to 60 percent of our total body weight is water? Water is our life force. In fact, we could only go a few days without water before our body would start to deteriorate and die. Every day our body uses water for all its internal cellular functions.

YOU ARE WHAT

YOU ARE

BY WHAT YOU

BELIEVE.

OPRAH

WINFREY

We lose about 64 ounces (1.9 litres) of water every day through cellular metabolism and perspiration. Cover your entire arm with a plastic bag, and within a few minutes you will get a very visual demonstration of how much water we lose in a day. Think of the good old-fashioned suits designed to make you sweat and lose weight. Yeah, you lost weight, but it was not fat weight; it was very valuable water weight. People who wore those sweat suits just became dehydrated.

The "eight glasses of water every day" prescription arose from the need to replenish the water that is lost every day through cellular respiration in all humans. Unfortunately, most people exist on a daily basis in a dehydrated state. Common complaints such as headaches, lack of energy, tired and lethargic sensations, and achy joints and muscles have all been associated with dehydration. If most people would commit to drinking eight glasses of water every day, they would notice a great improvement in their overall health and energy levels.

Think of it this way. Water is a component of every tissue cell, organ and system in your body, all of which function optimally only in the presence of adequate water levels. So even fat loss will not occur at an optimal rate if you are in a dehydrated state. If fat loss is to occur, the fat needs to be mobilized from the fat cell and released into the bloodstream to travel to muscle tissue to be used for energy. But the bloodstream has a high water content and will be unable to perform its job efficiently if the body is dehydrated. So water is also critical to fat loss.

My clients who have committed to ensuring they consume enough water every day have noticed a huge improvement in their fitness level and body composition. You will, too.

If you are an exerciser, different rules apply. In an hour of exercise, you might lose about 33 ounces (one litre) of water or more to help dissipate the heat that is being produced. So, if you exercise, you need to drink those eight glasses a day and, in addition, replenish the water you have lost during your workout. So follow this prescription: Drink water before exercise, during exercise, after exercise and anytime in between!

Take my word for it: water is definitely something that needs to be a priority. Here are two common questions I get from clients regarding water intake.

Every time I commit to drinking more water, I seem to spend all my time running to the washroom. Is there anything I can do about this? In the beginning, your body and its tissues are not used to absorbing this higher level of fluid, so they will just flush it out. And, yes, you will be spending a great deal of time in the restroom, but this will not last long. Eventually your body and its tissues will start to absorb the water, and your need to run to the washroom all day should decrease. Your body will soon adapt to your hydrated state. Your thirst mechanism will also become more efficient, and you will find that the more you drink, the more thirsty you become. That is a great sign!

Does it have to be water? I suggest that you consume at least eight glasses of good, wholesome, refreshing water every day. Any other additional fluids you consume in the form of juice, milk or herbal teas will be a bonus.

HOMEWORK

I'm sure you know that drinking water is very important, but I am going to guess that you're probably not adhering to the eight-glasses-per-day prescription. It is not enough to say you need to start drinking more water. We need to figure out how you are going to do this. For example, one of your goals might be to purchase a water bottle that you carry with you everywhere you go or to purchase bottled water from a water company so you always have cold water available. It is imperative that you figure out how you can commit to drinking the required amount of water.

List some action steps you can take to ensure you drink the required amount of water.

_____

_____

_____

_____

_____

_____

_____

_____

DESIGNING A REALISTIC EATING PLAN

"EAT AFTER EIGHT, YOU GAIN WEIGHT"

Eating habits play almost as big a part in weight gain as the calories you ingest. See if you recognize yourself in any of the following. You wake up in the morning full of determination that "today is going to be the day" you will start that diet and get control of your weight. So you skip breakfast, guzzle coffee all morning and then, practising great self-control, eat a tiny lunch. By mid-afternoon you are starving, so you grab a quick pick-me-up chocolate bar or muffin. By the time you get home, you are hungry and tired and ready for dinner. You stuff yourself at the dinner table, then snack all evening. You go to bed on a full stomach, feeling guilty, and tomorrow the cycle begins all over again.

This type of eating pattern is common and has your body working against you rather than for you. Many people who do not eat breakfast and consume only a very light lunch are tricked into believing that they are reducing their caloric intake when, in fact, they are setting themselves up for a snacking binge in the late afternoon, followed by an overload at dinner and into the evening. The result is just the opposite of what they intend: total calories consumed during the day end up being greater rather than fewer. And the scale gives them the bad news that they are gaining weight.

Our bodies are not very good at burning calories from a big meal, especially in the evening, when all our systems tend to slow down. Many of our evening calories, then, may be more likely to be stored as fat.

A HEALTHY

BODY IS

A GUEST-CHAMBER

FOR THE SOUL;

A SICK BODY IS A

PRISON.

FRANCIS

BACON

Your metabolism, the rate at which you burn calories for internal functions, is like an engine – the more often you give it fuel, the better it works. When you deprive your body of food, even for short periods of time, your metabolism automatically slows down in order to preserve energy. And a slowed metabolism makes it much more difficult to lose weight. It does not need to be this way. The good news is you can get your body to work for you instead of against you. The rule should be to go no more than four hours without eating something.

Think of starting your day with food as revving your internal engine. Regardless of whether you are a breakfast person or not, you must develop the habit of having something to eat in the morning. Your mom was right, breakfast is the most important meal of the day, but it does not need to be a five-course meal. A piece of fruit, a bagel, cereal and milk, or toast and juice will suffice. Then, a few hours later, have a small snack, such as a piece of fruit or a cup of yogurt. By lunchtime, you are not going to have a problem making a healthy, low-fat, low-calorie choice. A half-sandwich and salad or bowl of chili or vegetable soup might be an appropriate lunch. A few hours later, in the afternoon, eat another light snack, such as a few celery and carrot sticks or crackers and cheese. By the time dinner comes around, you will not be ravenous and you will be less likely to indulge and consume too many calories.

This type of eating pattern keeps your metabolism revving all day, keeps your energy level up and helps you avoid the tendency to overeat at any meal. Most of us have been conditioned to believe that dinner should be the largest meal of the day, so changing your eating patterns is not going to be easy. It will not happen overnight. You will probably have to change other old habits, too. If, for example, you snack in the evening while watching TV, you might need to go for a walk in the evening instead. If you find yourself bored in the evening and eating because there is nothing else to do, enroll in an evening course or start reading a good book. Breaking habits is very difficult in the beginning, but eventually the new habits become second nature.

HOMEWORK

In the following section, practise designing a full-day eating plan. Do not worry about whether the food items you include in each section are the "right" choices. Instead, focus on including the things you enjoy eating and that you believe would be healthy choices. We'll fine-tune your nutrition plan later.

What time could you normally consume a healthy breakfast? _____

List two or three healthy breakfasts you would consider enjoyable.

_____

_____

_____

What time could you normally consume a mid-morning snack? _____

List two or three healthy mid-morning snacks you would consider enjoyable.

_____

_____

_____

What time could you normally consume a healthy lunch? _____

List two or three healthy lunches you would consider enjoyable.

_____

_____

_____

What time could you normally consume a mid-afternoon snack? _____

List two or three healthy mid-afternoon snacks you would consider enjoyable.

_____

_____

_____

What time could you normally consume a healthy dinner? _____

List two or three healthy dinners you would consider enjoyable.

_____

_____

_____

YES, YOU CAN EAT CAKE!

A successful nutrition plan will focus on what you need to be consuming every day rather than what you should not be eating. For example, set a goal of eating three servings of fruit each day instead of deciding not to eat any chocolate. In addition, allow yourself one or two "free" days every week. For example, if you love pizza, wine and chocolate, then one day a week allow yourself to indulge in these items. This will eliminate the feeling of being deprived of your favourite foods, and you will be less likely to experience the inevitable binge that goes hand in hand with total elimination of your favourites.

This type of plan is feasible for most people. You are not telling yourself you are never going to eat chocolate again, but instead limiting how much you will eat and when you will indulge. Just make sure you do not start to make deals with yourself regarding your free days. If Saturday is your free day, make sure you stick to Saturday. Avoid indulging on, say, Thursday, then promising yourself that on Saturday you will skip your free day. These types of compromises can lead to others.

Do you ever wonder why you cannot seem to stop after one piece of chocolate? We know that simple sugars cause blood insulin levels to increase. High insulin levels stimulate

YOU
CANNOT
DIRECT
WHICH
WAY THE
WINDS OF
ADVERSITY
WILL BLOW,
BUT YOU
CAN
ADJUST
YOUR
SAILS.

SHANTIDASA

fat uptake by fat cells and inhibit fat use in muscle. This is one of the reasons complex carbohydrates (brown rice, whole wheat pasta and breads) are recommended compared to simple carbohydrates (sugars) to help maximize fat loss. We also know that eating fat stimulates our craving for more fat. This is why you should limit your free days to just one or two a week. This will help to avoid the innocent "I'll just have one" that turns into consuming the contents of the whole box or bag. Sometimes it is better to just hold off and demonstrate your ability to delay gratification.

I prefer to follow the 80/20 rule for nutrition, which states that if you are eating well 80 percent of the time, you can allow yourself to indulge the other 20 percent. Eating well 80 percent of the time will definitely get you to your fat loss goals and will be a much more enjoyable process. This philosophy is focused on the long term. It is important that you decide to only do things that you can see yourself doing for the rest of your life. The only way to do this is to achieve your goals while upsetting your life as little as possible.

HOMEWORK

Based on the information in the previous section and the goals set out in Your Fat Loss Contract, outline some nutrition goals you believe you can adhere to. For example, you might decide you will consume five small meals or snacks each day, drink five glasses of water each day, include one free day each week, consume three vegetable and three fruit servings each day or drink wine with dinner only two nights each week. Establish goals that are realistic for you. Remember, small changes often bring about significant differences to your health and body composition.

List the nutrition goals you feel you can adhere to on a long-term basis.

_____

_____

_____

_____

_____

_____

_____

_____

_____

_____

There are some foods you will definitely want to consume in limited quantities only on your free days. Here is the list.

- **Fried foods.** *During the cooking process, these foods soak up the oil like a sponge.*

- **Creams.** *These dairy products have a very high fat content.*

- **Processed foods.** *Always go for wholesome, fresh foods as the staples in your diet. They will always be higher in nutrients and lower in fat. Processed foods should only complement a diet that is rich in fresh fruits, vegetables and whole wheat grains.*

- **Alcohol.** *Although low in fat content, alcohol is very high in empty calories. In addition, alcohol activates the enzyme that takes up fat from our bloodstream and stores it in our fat cells. Therefore, any food we consume in combination with alcohol will more likely end up in our fat storage depot areas, such as our hips, thighs and stomach. And, finally, alcohol lowers our inhibitions, making us more likely to make poorer food choices.*

- **Caffeine.** *Limit your intake of drinks containing caffeine for the reasons outlined later in this chapter.*

- **No-fat products.** *You are probably thinking, "What? Limit no-fat foods? But aren't they the answer to all my fat loss prayers?" It is interesting to note that even with the explosion of no-fat products onto the market, our population continues to get fatter and fatter. You would think we would start to get skinnier as we consumed more of these no-fat products. But what makes those no-fat products taste so good? Sugar – and lots of it. And what is sugar made of? A lot of calories. Excess calories, whether they come from no-fat cookies or full-fat cookies, are still going to show up as fat on our hips and thighs and stomachs.*

> LIVE YOUR LIFE EACH DAY AS YOU WOULD CLIMB A MOUNTAIN. AN OCCASIONAL GLANCE TOWARD THE SUMMIT KEEPS THE GOAL IN MIND, BUT MANY BEAUTIFUL SCENES ARE TO BE OBSERVED FROM EACH NEW VANTAGE POINT.
>
> HAROLD V. MELCHERT

Here is a very important message to remember. If, at the end of the day, you have eaten excess calories from any source, you will store those calories as fat. Here is how it works. Let's say you consume an extra 1,000 carbohydrate calories in the form of plain pasta. It takes about 23 percent of the calories consumed to break down the dietary carbohydrate and store it as body fat. So, out of the 1,000 extra carbohydrate calories, 770 will be stored as body fat.

Now let's say you consume an extra 1,000 fat calories in the form of creams. It takes about three percent of the calories consumed to break down this dietary fat and store it as body fat. So, out of the 1,000 extra fat calories, 970 will be stored as body fat.

It is obviously better to be consuming a diet rich in carbohydrates, because less of the excess will be stored as body fat. But you will store excess carbohydrates as body fat and you will gain weight whether your diet is low in fat or not. If your diet contains more

A MAN IS

NOT OLD

UNTIL REGRETS

TAKE THE

PLACE OF

DREAMS.

JOHN

BARRYMORE

calories than you expend in a day, you will gain weight regardless of the source of the calories.

- **High-fat foods.** *Dietary fat is very easily converted to body fat. Limit any food choices that are higher than 30 percent fat content. Here is an easy formula to determine the fat content of your favourite foods.*

1. Read the label to determine the number of grams of fat per serving.

2. Multiply the number of grams of fat by nine to determine how many fat calories are in the food. (There are nine calories in one gram of fat.)

3. Read the label to determine the total number of calories in one serving. It's usually listed under the heading of "energy."

4. Now divide the number of fat calories by the total number of calories to determine the fat percentage. If the percentage is 30 or less, the food is low-fat.

HOMEWORK:

Go and grab 10 items out of your kitchen cupboard that you eat regularly and your calculator. Let's determine whether the items you picked are healthy choices or not.

SAMPLE ONE

Item: _____

Number of fat grams (from label): _____

Number of fat calories = number of fat grams (_____) x 9 = _____

Number of total calories (from label): _____

Fat percentage = Number of fat calories (_____) ÷ number of total calories (_____) x 100 = _____ %

Circle one: Healthy choice   Less healthy choice
                        (< 30%)   (> 30%)

S A M P L E TWO

Item: _____

Number of fat grams (from label): _____

Number of fat calories = number of fat grams (_____) x 9 = _____

Number of total calories (from label): _____

Fat percentage = Number of fat calories (_____) ÷ number of total calories (_____) x 100 = _____ %

Circle one: Healthy choice   Less healthy choice
                     (< 30%)   (> 30%)

S A M P L E THREE

Item: _____

Number of fat grams (from label): _____

Number of fat calories = number of fat grams (_____) x 9 = _____

Number of total calories (from label): _____

Fat percentage = Number of fat calories (_____) ÷ number of total calories (_____) x 100 = _____ %

Circle one: Healthy choice   Less healthy choice
                     (< 30%)   (> 30%)

S A M P L E FOUR

Item: _____

Number of fat grams (from label): _____

Number of fat calories = number of fat grams (_____) x 9 = _____

Number of total calories (from label): _____

Fat percentage = Number of fat calories (_____) ÷ number of total calories (_____) x 100 = _____ %

Circle one: Healthy choice   Less healthy choice
                     (< 30%)   (> 30%)

SAMPLE FIVE

Item: _____

Number of fat grams (from label): _____

Number of fat calories = number of fat grams (_____) x 9 = _____

Number of total calories (from label): _____

Fat percentage = Number of fat calories (_____) ÷ number of total calories (_____) x 100 = _____ %

Circle one: Healthy choice   Less healthy choice
                      (< 30%)   (> 30%)

SAMPLE SIX

Item: _____

Number of fat grams (from label): _____

Number of fat calories = number of fat grams (_____) x 9 = _____

Number of total calories (from label): _____

Fat percentage = Number of fat calories (_____) ÷ number of total calories (_____) x 100 = _____ %

Circle one: Healthy choice   Less healthy choice
                      (< 30%)   (> 30%)

SAMPLE SEVEN

Item: _____

Number of fat grams (from label): _____

Number of fat calories = number of fat grams (_____) x 9 = _____

Number of total calories (from label): _____

Fat percentage = Number of fat calories (_____) ÷ number of total calories (_____) x 100 = _____ %

Circle one: Healthy choice   Less healthy choice
                      (< 30%)   (> 30%)

SAMPLE EIGHT

Item: _____

Number of fat grams (from label): _____

Number of fat calories = number of fat grams (_____) x 9 = _____

Number of total calories (from label): _____

Fat percentage = Number of fat calories (_____) ÷ number of total calories (_____) x 100 = _____ %

Circle one: Healthy choice   Less healthy choice
                     (< 30%)   (> 30%)

SAMPLE NINE

Item: _____

Number of fat grams (from label): _____

Number of fat calories = number of fat grams (_____) x 9 = _____

Number of total calories (from label): _____

Fat percentage = Number of fat calories (_____) ÷ number of total calories (_____) x 100 = _____ %

Circle one: Healthy choice   Less healthy choice
                     (< 30%)   (> 30%)

SAMPLE TEN

Item: _____

Number of fat grams (from label): _____

Number of fat calories = number of fat grams (_____) x 9 = _____

Number of total calories (from label): _____

Fat percentage = Number of fat calories (_____) ÷ number of total calories (_____) x 100 = _____ %

Circle one: Healthy choice   Less healthy choice
                     (< 30%)   (> 30%)

While reading the labels, also look at the order of ingredients. If fat is listed as one of the first, second or third ingredients, the product is likely to he high in fat and is best avoided. Items such as lard, animal shortening, oil of any kind, butterfat, whole milk solids, shortening and margarine are all fats.

It is also wise to pay close attention to serving sizes listed on labels. Sometimes what is listed as one serving size is unrealistically small. So you might trick yourself into believing you are consuming an item that is low in calories and fat when what you are actually consuming is four times the listed serving size. It is also a good idea to choose products whose sugar content is less than 10 percent of the total carbohydrate content.

As you begin to reduce the amount of fat and increase the number of fruits and vegetables in your diet, your fibre intake will increase. You might notice that you start to experience a lot more intestinal gas when you start to adopt many of these healthy nutritional patterns. To reduce the initial negative effects of a high-fibre diet, change your diet gradually. Soon your body will adapt to your new, healthier diet.

SAY NO TO SUPERSIZE

We are victims of a society that is hooked on supersizing everything. We have supersize shakes and fries, monster-size cookies, muffins and bagels, and astronomical restaurant entrées. For many of us, it might not be our food choices that are poor; it might be that we are just eating too much of a good thing. Here is a chart based on Canada's Food Guide to help you determine the appropriate number of daily servings from each food group. Find the category you fit within.

DAILY SERVING REQUIREMENTS

	For most people	For people with active jobs (e.g., construction work) and for most athletes	For endurance athletes such as distance runners, cyclists and triathletes
Grain products	minimum 5 servings	8 servings or more	15 servings or more
Veggies & fruits	minimum 5 servings	8 servings or more	15 servings or more
Meats & alternatives	2 servings	2 servings	2 to 4 servings
Milk products	Adults: 2 servings; Children, teens, pregnant or lactating women: 3 to 4 servings	Adults: 2 servings; Children, teens, pregnant or lactating women: 3 to 4 servings	Adults: 2 to 6 servings; Children, teens, pregnant or lactating women: 3 to 6 servings

Now that you know how many servings you require from each food group, it is important to figure out the exact size of one serving. Here is another helpful chart.

SERVING SIZES

FOOD GROUP	ONE-SERVING SIZE EQUIVALENTS
Grains	• 1 slice of bread • 1/2 large bun, English muffin, bagel or pita • 1 small roll, biscuit or muffin • 4 to 6 crackers • 1/2 cup (125 mL) cooked rice or pasta • 1 ounce (30 g) of cold cereal • 1/2 cup (125 mL) of hot cereal
Veggies & fruits	• 1 medium-sized whole fruit or vegetable • 1/2 cup (125 mL) juice • 1/2 cup (125 mL) fresh, frozen or canned vegetables or fruit • 1 cup (250 mL) salad • 1/4 cup (50 mL) dried fruit
Meats & alternatives	• 3 ounces (50 to 100 g) cooked meat (size of a deck of cards) • 1 to 2 eggs • 1/2 to 1 cup (125 to 250 mL) beans or peas • 2 Tbsp. (30 mL) peanut butter • 1/3 to 2/3 can (50 to 100 g) fish • 1/3 cup (100 g) tofu
Milk products	• 1 cup (250 mL) milk • 2 ounces (50 g) cheese • 2 slices processed cheese • 3/4 cup (175 g) yogurt • 2 cups (500 mL) cottage cheese • 1 1/2 cups (375 mL) ice cream

1 cup = 250 mL   **1 Tbsp. = 15 mL**

EXERCISE,
EXERCISE YOUR
POWERS; WHAT IS
DIFFICULT WILL
FINALLY BECOME
ROUTINE.

GEORGE C.
LICHTENBERG

HOMEWORK

It is not enough to know the weight or volume of serving sizes. You should have a good understanding of the size of a serving in each of the food groups. For example, how much is one ounce (30 g) of cold cereal or two ounces (50 g) of cheese? The purpose of the following drill is to give you a visual picture of one serving size.

From your kitchen cupboards, pull out a variety of items from each of the four food groups. Now determine one serving size of each of the items using the above chart. Where possible, weigh or measure out individual servings.

By performing this drill, when it is time to prepare a meal you will know exactly how much food you need, and how much is too much.

REDUCING PORTION SIZES

When reducing food intake and portion sizes, the reduction should occur in the following order.

1. Reduce fat intake.

2. Reduce alcohol intake.

3. Reduce sugar intake.

4. Reduce starches (pasta, breads, rice).

To review, in combination with the above four suggestions, the most important nutritional habits to follow to maximize fat loss are these.

1. Drink adequate amounts of water.

2. Consume at least five vegetable servings and three fruit servings every day.

3. Eat five small meals or snacks each day.

4. Consume a diet that is 60 percent carbohydrates, 25 percent fat and 15 percent protein.

5. Avoid eating too late in the evening.

A NO-FAT DIET IS NOT HEALTHY

Fat has gotten a really bad rap. Although a reduction in dietary fat is usually a good thing, there is a point of diminishing returns and the possibility of health risks. Fat is the best fuel ever designed! We can make fat out of almost anything we eat. Can you imagine if your car could do that? Put in potatoes and the engine miraculously converts them into gas. In go hot dogs and instantly we get gasoline. Fat is an amazing fuel that provides us with a limitless amount of energy. Instead of hating fat and blaming it for all our problems, we should be astounded and respect it for its outstanding capabilities. Certain fatty acids are also necessary for good health, and certain "fat soluble" vitamins require fat for absorption into the system. Fat also helps to keep us insulated and warm.

Although most people need not worry about getting too little fat in their diet, there is another reason to be less obsessed about reducing fat to superlow levels: fat contributes to feelings of satiety and helps reduce food cravings. People who cut a lot of fat out of their diets often eat far too much of other "non-fat" foods that are high in calories. The key is to make sure that your total fat intake is within the accepted guidelines of 20 to 30 percent of total daily calories. No more than 10 percent of this should come from saturated fats (explanation to follow). The average fat content of most diets is greater than 43 percent. This is what is making our society fatter! The major sources of fat in our diets are dairy foods, including ice cream, spreads and sauces, so limit your intake of these items.

If you decide to set your fat intake to 25 percent of total daily calories, the total amount of fat you would need to consume, depending on your particular circumstance, is:

- *30 to 50 grams if you are a woman or a child*

- *40 to 60 grams if you are a man*

- *70 grams if you are a teenager or very active adult*

- *80 to 100 grams if your job requires heavy physical labour or if you are an endurance athlete*

- *30 to 40 grams if your goal is to lose body fat*

When deciding to reduce your fat intake, remember that there are fats in your diet that are obvious – foods such as butter, margarine, cooking oils and fat on meat. But there are also fats that are hidden in processed foods such as cakes, cookies and potato chips. It is important to limit your intake of fat from both these sources.

There are two basic classifications of fat: unsaturated (monounsaturated and polyunsaturated) and saturated. Unsaturated fats, especially the monounsaturated ones, are considered "healthier" and are found in nuts, seeds, vegetable oils and soft margarine products. Saturated fats are found in animal products such as beef, butter, dairy products and lard. They tend to raise blood cholesterol levels, thereby increasing the risk for heart disease.

> SELF-CONTROL MAY BE DEVELOPED, IN PRECISELY THE SAME MANNER AS WE TONE UP A WEAK MUSCLE - BY LITTLE EXERCISES DAY BY DAY.
>
> W.G. JORDAN

Also be cautious of consuming large amounts of coconut and palm oils. These are vegetable oils, but they contain a large amount of saturated fat. You might also have heard of transfatty acids. These are the end products of a process called hydrogenation, in which vegetable oils are hardened, and are found in products such as peanut butter. You should also limit your consumption of this type of fat.

HOMEWORK

List some easy ways you can reduce the amount of fat in your diet.

_____

_____

_____

_____

_____

_____

_____

_____

_____

CONTROLLING YOUR EATING ENVIRONMENT

When you are trying to adopt a healthier diet, your eating environment is also an important consideration. Some studies have found that we eat more when participating in other activities, like watching TV or studying, or when listening to fast music compared to slower music. Other studies have found we may make poorer choices when eating out with friends.

You need to consider your particular situation and personality and attempt to develop an environment that encourages slow eating and discourages overeating. We know that the brain requires 20 minutes to receive the signal that we are full. We have all probably experienced this phenomenon. For example, at Thanksgiving dinner, there was so much food and it all tasted so good that we gobbled it all down as quickly as possible. Fifteen minutes later we felt gross, bloated and knew we had eaten way too much. But at that point, there was nothing we could do about it. Had we eaten a little more slowly, our brain would have had the opportunity to send the message to stop eating.

FILLING THE CUPBOARDS AND FRIDGE

What happens if you get home and you are starved and there is nothing to eat? You are more likely to choose a less-healthy item or dial up a take-out restaurant and order something high in fat. If you want to commit to a healthy diet, you have to commit to setting up a framework for success. This includes planning a weekly trip to the grocery store and making a few smaller trips during the week to stock up on fresh fruits and veggies. You cannot expect to adhere to a healthy diet without making this very important commitment to yourself.

The time and day of the week I will commit to shopping to stock
my cupboards and fridge will be

_____

Cook-a-thons will also make sticking to your nutrition plan
a lot easier. Opening the fridge to find a bowl of chili, homemade
soup, pasta salad or chopped vegetables will make you more likely to grab for these healthier items. Spend one day a week preparing tasty food items you can quickly grab for lunch or dinner.

The time and day of the week I will commit to preparing food for
the upcoming week will be

_____

EATING ON THE GO

I can appreciate that sometimes life is so busy that it becomes
difficult to stick to a healthy eating plan. Here are some ideas for
those of you always on the go.

You must eat breakfast no matter how busy you are. Try these
balanced, quick breakfast options.

- *low-fat yogurt and some mixed raisins, granola and dried fruit*
- *cold or hot cereal with milk and fruit*
- *toast and fruit*
- *peanut butter and banana sandwich*
- *bagel with cream cheese and a piece of fruit*
- *homemade muffin and a banana*
- *fruit smoothie made from milk, yogurt and fruit*

Are you rushing to business meetings on your lunch?
Here are some easy lunch ideas to pack along or take out.

- *raw veggies with a container of plain yogurt for dipping*
- *sandwiches (tuna in pita bread or thick whole wheat bread, vegetables and cheese on a bagel, turkey and vegetables in pita bread, ricotta cheese and jam on your favourite bread, hummus and tomato on a baguette, cottage cheese and pineapple on a kaiser bun)*
- *pita pizzas with vegetables and tomato sauce*
- *low-fat crackers and cheese*
- *leftovers from dinner*
- *soup or chili made on the weekend*
- *baked potato with low-fat sour cream*
- *pasta salad made on the weekend*

> I WAS NEVER
> IN A HURRY
> IN MY LIFE.
> HE LIVES LONG
> WHO ENJOYS
> LIFE AND BEARS
> NO JEALOUSY
> OF OTHERS,
> WHOSE HEART
> HARBOURS NO
> MALICE OR ANGER,
> WHO SINGS
> A LOT AND CRIES
> A LITTLE, WHO
> RISES AND
> RETIRES WITH
> THE SUN, WHO
> LIKES TO WORK,
> AND WHO KNOWS
> HOW TO REST.
>
> SHIRALI
> MISLIMOV

PERSEVERANCE
IS A GREAT
ELEMENT OF
SUCCESS. IF
YOU ONLY
KNOCK
LONG ENOUGH
AND LOUD
ENOUGH AT
THE GATE, YOU
ARE SURE
TO WAKE UP
SOMEBODY.

HENRY W.
LONGFELLOW

Need a quick pick-me-up? Be sure to have a mid-morning and a mid-afternoon, low-fat, high-energy snack. Here are some healthy choices.

- *low-fat yogurt and fruit*
- *raw vegetables and yogurt dip*
- *fruit and yogurt dip*
- *PowerBar or Harvest energy bar*
- *glass of juice or milk*
- *hard-boiled egg*
- *low-fat crackers and cheese*
- *couple of fig bars*

CHEQUE, PLEASE

One study found that 88 percent of women ate away from home at least one out of four days. Another study found that consumers spend over $149 billion dollars at restaurants. That is a lot of eating out! So how do you stay on track when you do not have control of food preparation? Just remember that you actually do have control. When eating out, practise the following healthy behaviours.

- *Order water immediately.*
- *Order butter and salad dressing on the side.*
- *Ask for your meat broiled and without any additional fat added.*
- *Ask for your chicken to be prepared without the skin.*
- *Order a salad instead of french fries.*
- *Ask for skim milk.*
- *Order a tomato instead of a cream sauce for pasta dishes.*
- *Order plain bread instead of garlic bread.*
- *Take one piece of bread from the basket, then ask for the basket to be taken away.*
- *Order tomato and broth soups instead of cream-based soups.*
- *Order fresh fruit desserts.*
- *Hold the sauce on burgers and instead use ketchup, mustard, relish, tomato and lettuce.*
- *Do not be afraid to ask for any type of substitution.*

List restaurants that offer healthy choices that you could start going to.

_____

_____

_____

_____

_____

List some actions you can take to make better choices when you do eat out.

_____

_____

_____

_____

_____

_____

_____

_____

_____

_____

_____

_____

CHEMICAL PITFALLS

Despite all my pleadings, many of you might still be tempted by "get-thin-quick" schemes. I hope the following will convince you to stay away from these money traps.

Diet pills. The main ingredient of many of these is the stimulant phenylpropanolamine (PPA). When PPA is taken in large does, its effects resemble those of amphetamines or "speed." In low does, PPA immediately constricts blood vessels and speeds the heart rate, resulting in an acute elevation of blood pressure. Other potential side effects are anxiety, insomnia, headaches, irregular heart rhythms and the possibility of strokes or seizures.

Fat-burning enzymes. We know that in order to mobilize and utilize fat, certain fat-burning enzymes are required. As you can imagine, individuals looking for a get-rich-quick scheme have started to sell bottled enzymes. Unfortunately, these are a fraud. As soon as these enzymes hit your stomach acids, they are attacked, broken apart and incapacitated. Do not be fooled into wasting your money. The only way to build more fat-burning enzymes is to exercise regularly.

THE FIRST
STEP IS WHAT
COUNTS: FIRST
BEGINNINGS
ARE HARDEST
TO MAKE AND
AS SMALL AND
INCONSPICUOUS
AS THEY ARE POTENT
IN INFLUENCE,
BUT ONCE THEY
ARE MADE, IT IS
EASY TO ADD
THE REST.

ARISTOTLE

Pyruvate, creatine, chromium picolinate. For as long as people struggle with weight loss, there are always going to be manufacturers of the next magical fat loss pill. You can purchase literally hundreds of different products claiming to maximize fat loss. Unfortunately, no studies have proven any of the claims to be true. So, at the risk of sounding like a broken record, I repeat that the only proven way to shed those extra fat pounds is to exercise and eat well.

Caffeine. You might have heard that caffeine stimulates the release of fatty acids, and yes, this is true. However, this has led many to mistakenly believe that drinking coffee will speed fat loss. Perhaps this is one of the reasons for the success of the Starbucks chain! Before you start stocking up on extra coffee beans, let me explain why, in reality, drinking coffee will not make you thinner. The most obvious evidence is the average coffee drinker. Most North Americans drink a lot of coffee, and if caffeine speeds up fat loss, you would expect us to be a pretty thin population. But this is not the case. Although caffeine may stimulate the release of fatty acids into the bloodstream, if the muscles do not need the fat, the fat is sent right back home to the fat cell.

And caffeine has its own problems. Caffeine is a very powerful drug with quick, noticeable and measurable effects on the central nervous system, peripheral nervous system and digestive system. It is used in many prescription and over-the-counter pills. Like other drugs, it is habit-forming, and users find they have to have more and more caffeine to get the same effects. Caffeine makes a lot of people nervous, jittery and tense. It can often lead to bowel irritation and diarrhea. It is a diuretic and thus promotes water loss from the body. Treat caffeine as you would alcohol – a little bit once in a while is okay. Moderation is the key! Stick to one or two small cups of coffee or tea a day.

VITAMINS, MINERALS AND ANTIOXIDANTS

As a supplement to a healthy diet, I recommend you take one multivitamin every day. Choose one that offers close to 100 percent of the required dosage of as many vitamins and minerals as possible. You might also want to consider taking a calcium-magnesium supplement. And, finally, an antioxidant pill is also recommended. These are the only pills that I believe are necessary to maintain health and maximize fat loss.

HOMEWORK

We have covered a lot of material in this chapter, and now it is time to put it to good use. Your homework is to design a sample weeklong healthy nutrition plan based on everything you have learned in this chapter. Use the following charts to create your nutrition plan.

HEALTHY NUTRITIION

DAY: _____

	TIME OF DAY	FOOD CHOICES AND PORTION SIZES	WATER INTAKE
Breakfast			
Mid-morning snack			
Lunch			
Mid-afternoon snack			
Dinner			

CHECKS AND BALANCES:

Have you planned to consume eight glasses of water?

Have you planned to consume five vegetable and three fruit servings?

Have you planned to consume five small meals and snacks?

Have you avoided foods that are high in fat, salt, sugar and alcohol?

Have you planned a diet that is 60 percent carbohydrate, 25 percent fat and 15 percent protein?

Have you planned for portion sizes that are appropriate for your needs?

HEALTHY NUTRITIION

DAY: _____

	TIME OF DAY	FOOD CHOICES AND PORTION SIZES	WATER INTAKE
Breakfast			
Mid-morning snack			
Lunch			
Mid-afternoon snack			
Dinner			

CHECKS AND BALANCES:

Have you planned to consume eight glasses of water?

Have you planned to consume five vegetable and three fruit servings?

Have you planned to consume five small meals and snacks?

Have you avoided foods that are high in fat, salt, sugar and alcohol?

Have you planned a diet that is 60 percent carbohydrate, 25 percent fat and 15 percent protein?

Have you planned for portion sizes that are appropriate for your needs?

HEALTHY
NUTRITIION

DAY: _____

	TIME OF DAY	FOOD CHOICES AND PORTION SIZES	WATER INTAKE
Breakfast			
Mid-morning snack			
Lunch			
Mid-afternoon snack			
Dinner			

CHECKS AND BALANCES:

Have you planned to consume eight glasses of water?

Have you planned to consume five vegetable and three fruit servings?

Have you planned to consume five small meals and snacks?

Have you avoided foods that are high in fat, salt, sugar and alcohol?

Have you planned a diet that is 60 percent carbohydrate, 25 percent fat and 15 percent protein?

Have you planned for portion sizes that are appropriate for your needs?

HEALTHY NUTRITIION

DAY: _____

	TIME OF DAY	FOOD CHOICES AND PORTION SIZES	WATER INTAKE
Breakfast			
Mid-morning snack			
Lunch			
Mid-afternoon snack			
Dinner			

CHECKS AND BALANCES:

Have you planned to consume eight glasses of water?

Have you planned to consume five vegetable and three fruit servings?

Have you planned to consume five small meals and snacks?

Have you avoided foods that are high in fat, salt, sugar and alcohol?

Have you planned a diet that is 60 percent carbohydrate, 25 percent fat and 15 percent protein?

Have you planned for portion sizes that are appropriate for your needs?

HEALTHY NUTRITIION

DAY: _____

	TIME OF DAY	FOOD CHOICES AND PORTION SIZES	WATER INTAKE
Breakfast			
Mid-morning snack			
Lunch			
Mid-afternoon snack			
Dinner			

CHECKS AND BALANCES:

Have you planned to consume eight glasses of water?

Have you planned to consume five vegetable and three fruit servings?

Have you planned to consume five small meals and snacks?

Have you avoided foods that are high in fat, salt, sugar and alcohol?

Have you planned a diet that is 60 percent carbohydrate, 25 percent fat and 15 percent protein?

Have you planned for portion sizes that are appropriate for your needs?

HEALTHY
NUTRITIION

DAY: _____

	TIME OF DAY	FOOD CHOICES AND PORTION SIZES	WATER INTAKE
Breakfast			
Mid-morning snack			
Lunch			
Mid-afternoon snack			
Dinner			

CHECKS AND BALANCES:

Have you planned to consume eight glasses of water?

Have you planned to consume five vegetable and three fruit servings?

Have you planned to consume five small meals and snacks?

Have you avoided foods that are high in fat, salt, sugar and alcohol?

Have you planned a diet that is 60 percent carbohydrate, 25 percent fat and 15 percent protein?

Have you planned for portion sizes that are appropriate for your needs?

HEALTHY NUTRIITON

DAY: _____

	TIME OF DAY	FOOD CHOICES AND PORTION SIZES	WATER INTAKE
Breakfast			
Mid-morning snack			
Lunch			
Mid-afternoon snack			
Dinner			

CHECKS AND BALANCES:

Have you planned to consume eight glasses of water?

Have you planned to consume five vegetable and three fruit servings?

Have you planned to consume five small meals and snacks?

Have you avoided foods that are high in fat, salt, sugar and alcohol?

Have you planned a diet that is 60 percent carbohydrate, 25 percent fat and 15 percent protein?

Have you planned for portion sizes that are appropriate for your needs?

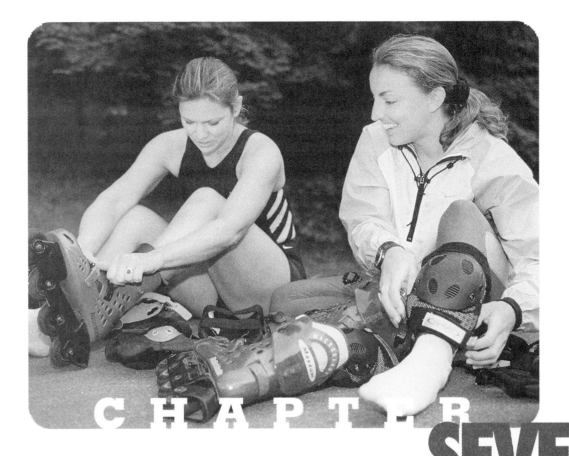

CHAPTER SEVEN

EXERCISING WITHOUT EXERCISING

Lack of time is the number one reason people say they cannot participate in an exercise program. But exercise does not need to involve a large time commitment. Just being active throughout the day means you do not have to spend hours at the gym. The problem is we have simply become too sedentary. The age of technology is making us fat. Escalators, elevators, remote controls, garage door openers, computers, home banking, the Internet, Takeout Taxi . . . We never have to leave the house. Things have gotten so bad that someone has invented an indoor treadmill for dogs so you do not even have to leave the couch to walk Spot!

Here are some ways to increase your daily caloric expenditure without actually "exercising."

- *Park one or two blocks away from wherever you are going and walk there.*
- *Walk or cycle if your destination is less than 20 minutes away.*
- *Always park in the farthest parking stall instead of hunting for the perfect spot right in front of the shop.*
- *Take the stairs if you need to go fewer than five flights.*
- *Take a 10-minute walk before work, at lunch or after dinner.*

- *Schedule active outings with your family or friends (hiking, cycling, walking, swimming, kayaking, indoor rock climbing).*
- *Do a few knee bends, heel raises or toe taps while making dinner.*
- *Do a few light exercises during TV commercials.*
- *At work, get up, move and stretch every 30 minutes. (Your back will thank you for it.)*
- *Sign up for a course (gardening, ballroom dancing, pottery). It will keep you busy and get you out of the house.*

One study at the University of South Carolina found that we expend approximately 10 fewer calories per day as a result of just using remote controls. Ten calories less – it does not sound like a lot. But by regularly using a remote control you are conceivably gaining one pound of fat per year! It is easy to see how people are putting weight on so easily and so quickly. In this day and age, it is a lot easier to eat 3,500 excess calories than it is to expend 3,500 calories.

If you are exercising three hours per week, what are you doing the other 165 hours? How you spend the time outside of your exercise sessions will make a huge difference to your fat loss efforts. Being active throughout the day will not take up any more of your time, but you will end up burning more calories and feeling a lot better.

HOMEWORK

List things you can commit to doing to increase your caloric expenditure throughout the day without actually exercising.

_____

_____

_____

_____

_____

_____

_____

_____

EXERCISE SHOULD NOT BE EXHAUSTING

Many exercisers make the mistake of working out so hard that when they are finished, they are completely exhausted. They often go home and take a nap or reduce their overall activity for the day so that by the end of the day, they might have burned the same amount of calories they would have had they not exercised at all. We want exercise to rejuvenate us, not tire us out. If you find you are too tired to take the stairs or walk to perform errands, or if you find yourself regularly needing sleep after workouts, you might be exercising too hard.

Many of us travel frequently for business purposes. Travelling without a plan can really sabotage any fat loss efforts. Here are some tips you can follow to ensure that travelling does not get in the way of your health and fitness goals.

Plan ahead. When flying, arrange with your airline for a healthy, low-fat, low-calorie meal. I always find the special meals much tastier, too. Bring your own water bottle and a few healthy snacks so you do not have to rely on the flight attendant's schedule for your own needs. When looking for a hotel, be sure to book with one that offers a hotel health club.

Keep moving. While flying, be sure to get up regularly and walk around at least every 30 minutes to enhance blood flow and minimize muscular and joint stiffness. Drink lots of water and avoid alcohol to help maintain your hydration levels.

Be on time. If switching time zones, adjust your watch to your destination time as soon as you get on the plane. Some studies have shown this will help you to adjust and will minimize jet lag.

Work out on arrival. If the timing is appropriate, do a light, low-intensity workout when you arrive at your destination. Recently I had to fly to Germany after having just completed a more than 20-hour flight from Australia to Vancouver, which meant a break of less than 24 hours before the second, 10-hour flight to Europe. I was exhausted and suffering from extreme jet lag. My body did not know what time it was. When I arrived in Germany it was 4:00 p.m. and all I wanted to do was sleep. But I forced myself to do a light, 30-minute run-walk, and when I was finished, I felt like a million bucks. Any signs of exhaustion had disappeared. The workout really helped me to adjust to my new time zone. Energy always seems to produce more energy. The workout does not have to be and should not be intense. A light workout to wake up your body is all you need.

Eat for energy. As soon as you can, find a local market and stock up on high-energy snacks like fruit, yogurt, energy bars and bottled water. Keep these items with you or chilled in your hotel room so you can continue consuming five small meals or snacks each day even though you are not following your regular routine. Whenever I travel, I carry a few PowerBars in my briefcase for those situations when I just can't seem to get away to grab something to eat. They're healthy, durable and fit nicely into a side pocket.

Watch your diet. When eating out, order water as soon as you sit down. Do not be afraid to make special requests. Ask about ingredients, preparation methods, portion size or substitutions, and be sure to request alternatives to create the healthy dinner you want. Be sure you stress the importance of your requests. If you must eat fast food, it does not necessarily need to be unhealthy. Stay away from fried foods like french fries, fried chicken or fried burgers. They are saturated with fat. Some pizzas may be a healthy choice. The crust is high in carbohydrates, the tomato sauce has no fat and the cheese is made from part-skim-milk mozzarella. Stick to all-veggie pizzas and avoid ordering extra cheese. Sandwiches or wraps minus the mayo are another healthy choice. Wendy's restaurants offer excellent healthy fast-food options such as chili, baked potatoes or grilled chicken sandwiches. Even a grilled hamburger (without the processed cheese) can be part of a healthy lunch. Just remember to commit to eating five small meals or snacks throughout the day. If you get too busy to eat, you will be more likely to make poor food choices.

Getting a massage is one of my favourite things. I have always dreamed that if I ever got rich enough, I would hire a live-in masseuse and I would start and finish every day with an hour-long massage. Heaven!

I encourage you to invest in a weekly massage, however, I do want to clear up any misconceptions regarding massage and its role in fat loss. Some massage therapists actually claim that massage helps with fat loss. Fat can only be mobilized, utilized and burned by muscles. It cannot be rubbed, massaged, kneaded or pounded away. Do you remember those old-fashioned exercise machines on which people sat on rollers in an attempt to "roll away" fat? Or the machines with the belt that were supposed to "shake off" fat? Both kinds of machines were humiliating and completely ineffective. The myth behind the massage and fat loss relationship is that the massage will loosen up fat so you can burn it more easily. This does not happen, and even if fat were "loosened up," it would be released from the fat cells and would travel to the muscles to be used. But since the muscles would not be doing anything, the fat would just turn around and find another fat cell to settle into.

FINDING A BALANCE

Achieving a healthy lifestyle is about a lot more than just exercise and a nutritious diet. Your program should allow for enough time to develop relationships with family and friends and time to participate in your favourite relaxing, stress-reducing activities, like reading, taking baths, watching sunsets, going to the movies, shopping or sleeping.

The following manifesto sums up my attitude toward finding balance in life. It is not just about reaching your fat loss goals. You have to enjoy the journey.

If I had my life to live over again, I'd dare to make more mistakes next time. I'd relax. I'd limber up. I'd be sillier than I've been this trip. I would take fewer things seriously. I would take more chances, I would take more trips, I would climb more mountains and swim more rivers. I would eat more ice cream and less beans. I would, perhaps, have more actual troubles but fewer imaginary ones. You see, I'm one of those people who was sensible and sane, hour after hour, day after day.

Oh, I've had my moments. If I had it to do over again, I'd have more of them. In fact, I'd try not to have anything else — just moments, one after another, instead of living so many years ahead of each day. I've been one of the persons who never goes anywhere without a thermometer, a hot-water bottle, a raincoat and a parachute. If I could do it again, I would travel lighter than I have.

If I had my life to live over, I would start barefoot earlier in the spring, and stay that way later in the fall. I would go to more dances, I would ride more merry-go-rounds, I would pick more daisies.

This poem was written by Nadine Stair, an 86-year-old woman, wishing she had done things a little differently. Don't wait until it is too late to enjoy life!

HOMEWORK

Outline the activities you want to do regularly to take care of yourself, so that when your time is up you will feel satisfied that you have lived a happy, fulfilled life.

_____

_____

_____

_____

_____

_____

_____

_____

_____

_____

_____

_____

_____

_____

_____

_____

_____

_____

_____

_____

_____

_____

_____

> REJOICE IN YOUR STRENGTH, REJOICE IN YOUR TALENTS AND POWERS, REJOICE IN THE WONDERS OF YOUR OWN NATURE. FOR THERE IS FAR MORE IN YOU THAN YOU EVER DREAMED.
>
> **CHRISTIAN D. LARSON**

Remember that your tombstone will give the date you were born and the date you died, with a dash in between. That dash – this interval – represents your life. You have the choice right now as to the type of life you will live. You could choose to become an unhealthy, crippled senior confined to a wheelchair, spending your last days in a nursing home. Or you could choose to exercise and eat well and enjoy your health into your later years. You could choose to be a highly stressed business executive running from appointment to appointment, deadline to deadline, fuelled by caffeine, fast foods and adrenaline until your body can't keep up. Or you could choose to be a lethargic soap opera fanatic with the only excitement in your life being who's sleeping with whom from noon to 5:00 p.m.

Very few people die and regret not having spent more time at the office, watching television or performing household chores. Instead they often wish they had spent more time with loved ones, taken bigger risks, been involved with more fun, exciting activities and learned to appreciate the beauty that surrounds us every day. Seize the day!

> YOU
> CANNOT
> LIVE YOUR
> DREAMS
> WHILE
> SITTING
> ON THE
> EASY
> CHAIR AT
> HOME.
>
> ROBERT S.
> MACDOUGALL
>
> •

Let's imagine this scenario. You have scheduled a two-week vacation and have decided to drive to your favourite holiday destination. You get halfway there, get a flat tire, get frustrated, and turn around and go back home. Would you actually turn around and go home? No, but that is what most people do who initiate an exercise or nutrition plan. They get off track, get discouraged and go back to their old habits and patterns. Why wouldn't they just fix the flat and keep on going to their destination? This is what you need to do. Accept that there are going to be some obstacles, challenges or perceived failures on your journey. But never lose sight of your destination. Use this book as a resource. You might find it helpful to refer to it every few months for inspiration if you start to lose your motivation. If you stumble, fix the flat and get back on track. Commit to staying fit – and believe in yourself!